The Joy of Healthy Living

The Guide To Eating Right For Life

Deborah Francis

Always Consult Your Physician First. Although it is helpful to get health information by reading and talking with friends, make sure you consult your doctor first before beginning any new treatment or changing your diet. Remember that the U.S. Food and Drug Administration do not strictly regulate the strength, purity or safety of herbs and supplements. Be sure to always read product labels. If you have a medical condition, or are taking other drugs, herbs, or supplements, speak with your doctor before taking medical action or changing your health routine. This information is not intended to replace the advice of a doctor. The Joy of Healthy Living LLC and Deborah Francis disclaim any liability for the decisions made by its readers based on the information provided.

The Joy of Healthy Living; The Guide To Eating Right For Life
Authors: Deborah Francis
Cover designed by: BTP Marketing Group
Edited By: BTP Marketing Group
ISBN: 978-0615635682

Published by: BTP Publishing Group, Plymouth, Fl

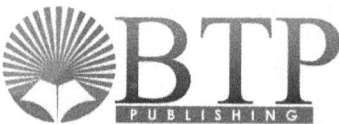

Also by Deborah Francis:

Built To Prosper For Women

Built To Prosper Financially

Built To Prosper Women of Wisdom Journal

Undeniable Confidence

CASHOLOGY

CASHOLOGY Wealth Workbook

CASHOLOGY Wealth Journal

Seminars by Deborah Francis

Built To Prosper For Life Seminars

CASHOLOGY Academy

Meet Deborah online and receive free training at

www.DeborahFrancisCompanies.com

www.BuiltToProsperCompanies.com

Table of Content

Fruit and Vegetable Prevention and Solutions to Common Disease and Illness

A

ACNE
apricots
cranberries
garlic
potatoes

ALLERGIES
apples

ANMEMIA
apricots
tomatoes

ANGINA
berries
cherries
oranges

ARTHRITIS
apples
garlic
mushrooms
potatoes

ASTHMA
bell peppers
oranges

B

BACTERIAL INFECTIONS
berries
cherries

carrots

garlic

BLADDER PROBLEMS

apples

berries

cherries

BLOOD CLEANSING

romaine lettuce

avocados

tomatoes

cucumbers

celery

carrots

red beets

zucchini

bell peppers

broccoli

cauliflower

cabbage

asparagus

onions

corn

potatoes

sweet potatoes

squash

watermelon

cantaloupe

pears

apples

bananas

mangoes

peaches

plums

nectarines
grapes
coconut
orange
grapefruit
berries

BLOOD CLOTS
mushrooms
pineapple

BLOOD PRESSURE
apples
garlic

BLOOD SUGAR
berries
cantaloupe
tomatoes
kale
Spinach
bell pepper
Brussels sprouts
cabbage
carrots

BLOOD VESSELS
berries
cherries

BOILS
potatoes

BRONCHITIS
bell peppers
garlic
oranges

BRUISES

potatoes

C

CANCER

avocados
bell peppers
berries
cherries
carrots
garlic
mushrooms
oranges
spinach
sweet potatoes
tomatoes
cabbage
kale

CARDIOVASCULAR

garlic
berries
cherries
grapes

CATARACTS

avocados
bell peppers
oranges
spinach

CHEST CONGESTION

garlic

CHOLESTEROL

avocados

bananas
blueberries
carrots
garlic
mushrooms
oranges

CIRCULATION

berries
cherries

COLDS

apples
lemons
oranges
grapefruit
berries
garlic
onion
mushrooms

CONSTIPATION

prunes
apples
bananas
avocados
carrots

CORNS

pineapples
bananas
apricots

COUGH

berries

cherries

garlic

CUTS

garlic

CYSTITIS

apple

cranberries

D

DEHYDRATION

water

watermelon

DEPPRESSION

potatoes

spinach

bananas

berries

cherries

DETOXIFICATION

romaine lettuce

avocados

tomatoes

cucumbers

celery

carrots

red beets

zucchini

bell peppers

broccoli

cauliflower

cabbage

asparagus

onions

corn
potatoes
sweet potatoes
squash
watermelon
cantaloupe
pears
apples
bananas
mangoes
peaches
plums
nectarines
grapes
coconut
orange
grapefruit
berries

DIABETES

berries
cantaloupe
tomatoes
kale
spinach
cabbage
carrots

DIARRHEA

bananas
berries
cherries
carrots

DIGESTION
pineapple

F

FATIGUE
apples
bananas

FEVER
bananas

FLU
garlic

FOOD POISONING
bananas
apples

FUNGAL INFECTION
garlic

G

GALLSTONES
potatoes

GOUT
berries
cherries
potatoes

GUMS
bell peppers
oranges

H

HAIR

apple

avocados

HAY FEVER

apples

oranges

grapes

tomatoes

HEADACHE

apple

potatoes

broccoli

kale

spinach

HEART

garlic

broccoli

onion

tomatoes

avocados

HEMORROIDS

apples

artichokes

avocados

beans

berries

broccoli

pears

squash

peas

I

IMMUNE SYSTEM

berries
cherries
carrots
garlic
mushrooms

Oranges
grapefruit
cantaloupe
spinach
broccoli
carrots
bell peppers
cauliflower
sweet potatoes

INFECTION
apple
garlic
berries
cherries
potatoes
onion

INSECT BITES
bananas
garlic

K

KIDNEY HEALTH
Red bell peppers
cabbage
cauliflower
garlic
onion
apples

cranberries
blueberries
strawberries
cherries
grapes

L

LARANGYITIS

pineapple
lemon
carrot juice
apricots
cantaloupe
orange
grapefruit
lime
cranberries

LONGEVITY

berries
cherries
pineapple
spinach
red bell   pepper
broccoli
tomatoes
apple
artichoke
arugula
asparagus
avocado
squash
cantaloupe
carrot

cauliflower
cabbage
kale
mango
mushroom
orange
watermelon

LUNGS

oranges
mushrooms
onions

M

MACULAR DEGENERATION

bell peppers
berries
carrots
spinach

MENTAL ALERTNESS

berries

MOOD ENHANCERS

potatoes
spinach

MUSCLES

bananas

O

OSTEOPOROSIS

pineapple

R

RELAXATION

spinach
broccoli
strawberry
figs
cherries
oranges
mangoes
pineapple
berries
grapefruit
bananas

RESPIRATORTY HEALTH

bell peppers
berries
cherries
oranges

S

SINUSES

apples
garlic

SKIN HEALTH

berries
cherries
grapes
cranberries
cabbage
kale
broccoli
garlic

SORE THROAT

garlic
bananas

oranges

mangoes

apples

STOMACHACHE

beans

grapes

grape fruit

apples

oranges

STROKE

mushroom

potatoes

SUNBURN

tomatoes

beans

mango

papaya

sweet potato

squash

carrot

SWELLING

pineapple

potato

apricots

bananas

broccoli

cantaloupe

carrots

mushrooms

oranges

parsnip

T

TEETH
melons
pears
celery
cucumbers

TENDINITIS
pineapple

TOOTHACHE
onion
garlic

U

ULCERS
bananas
apples
oranges
prunes
bananas
blueberries
pears
broccoli
sweet potatoes
cherries
spinach
kale

V

VIRUSES
berries
cherries
garlic

mushrooms
oranges

VISION
berries
carrots
kale
spinach
Squash
grapes

FOREWORD

When Deborah asked me to write the foreword to *The Joy of Healthy Living*, I was honored and excited. During the last several years, Deborah and I have talked on a regular basis about the subject of healthy living including: eating more fruits and vegetables; diet, exercise, plant based foods, natural living and so much more.

In fact, Deborah has exposed me to a health & wellness business opportunity that promotes a healthy lifestyle based on the consciousness of adding more fruits and vegetables to your diet on a daily basis. After joining Deborah's team, my knowledge of eating more fruits and vegetables along with taking whole food supplements has increased dramatically.

Furthermore, after joining Deborah's health & wellness virtual business team, I was inspired to continue promoting healthy living, by adding more fruits & vegetables to the menus at my Child Care Center and I write more about the healing powers of food in my blogs, *Natural Living 101* and *TheFabulousWoman.Wordpress.Com*.

Deborah has inspired me to transition from drinking animal based milk to drinking plant based milk. I must say that, after reading the information that Deborah has provided for me on plant based milk, I now prefer and enjoy drinking plant based milk regularly.

So to recommend this book allows me to introduce Deborah Francis and her health & wellness teaching and what better book to recommend than *The Joy of Healthy Living*.

As I reviewed the Introduction of this book, I could hardly wait to read the secrets revealed through out and I must say that you are in for a "Healthy" treat.

The Joy of Healthy Living will teach you how to use food as your medicine, choose foods that help to fight anxiety and depression; provide you with solutions for health and nutrition in prevention and recovery from cancer, heart disease, hypertension, diabetes and so much more.

Deborah has played a vital role in the transformation of my mindset about health & wellness and I believe that she will have that same affect on you as you read *The Joy of Healthy Living*.

Shiketa A. Morgan
Business Owner, Web Entrepreneur, Author, Editor at TheNaturalWayofLiving101.com.

Solutions available in this book to your most pressing questions about health.

How you can use food as medicine.

Is organic really better?

What foods fight anxiety and depression?

What are natural therapies for system based diseases?

What solutions are available for health using nutrition against cancer, heart disease, hypertension, diabetes, and more?

What foods do we need to eat for healthy aging?

What functional foods have health-promoting phytonutrients and antioxidant power?

How to overcome food allergies and intolerances?

What are low glycemic index foods?

How to choose the right foods for high performance and sports?

What to feed children with guidance on high performance based on nutrition from fruits and vegetables?

And more!

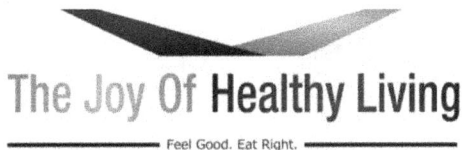

The Joy Of **Healthy Living**
Feel Good. Eat Right.

INTRODUCTION

An ounce of prevention is double the worth an ounce of cure.

"Let thy food be thy medicine, and thy medicine be thy food. ~
Hippocrates

During the time before pharmaceutical grade drugs came into effect many people across the world were known to cure themselves by the food they ate. Today, many make fun of the notion; thinking nutrition and medicine have little in common. Food has been reduced for many as a product to satisfy hunger while turning to pharmaceutical drugs to treat illness.

Another quote by Hippocrates, which is part of the Hippocratic Oath still recited by modern doctors today, is *"First, do no harm."*

Unfortunately, the obsession with the idea that there must be "a pill for every ill" now greatly compromises this oath, because the practice of medicine is primarily focused on drugs that often do far more harm than good. Meanwhile, modern doctors receive virtually little to no training in nutrition.

Turning our backs on the fundamental truth that "food is medicine" is no doubt at the heart of current disease epidemics. Negative changes in lifestyle and dietary patterns have resulted in modern world illnesses like coronary artery disease, diabetes, stroke, and cancer in higher frequency than ever before. Several research and experimental studies have clearly suggested that the trends in disease patterns are clearly linked to the diet we consume. Consequently, new interest has prompted a greater awareness in the synergistic medicinal qualities of fruits and vegetables.

What is the Big ORGANIC Deal?

Here is a brief assortment of the benefits of eating organically:

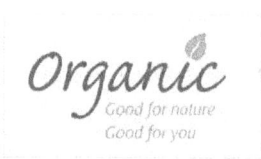

Organic Good for nature Good for you — Organic produce has higher levels of beneficial antioxidants and phytonutrients.

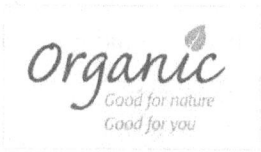

Organic Good for nature Good for you — No pesticide, herbicide, fungicide residues on food.

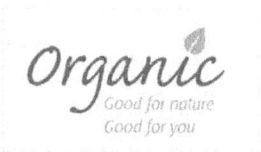

Organic Good for nature Good for you — No synthetic fertilizer residuals built into plants.

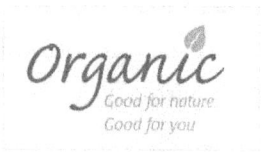

Organic Good for nature Good for you — No genetically engineered organisms or varieties.

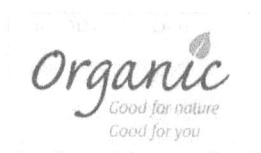

Organic Good for nature Good for you — Intense, realistic flavors. Higher vitamin and mineral variety and content

When looking at food and nutrition it is imperative to understand what happens to the nutrient content of food when it is processed, and the potential harm that can be caused by added chemicals. Our food stores are packed with processed foods that not only contain ingredients grown in exhausted pesticide-laden soils to begin with, but are further depleted of real nutrients through processing; in the end providing hardly anything beyond empty calories.

According to the Organic Consumers Association, the (12 most pesticide-laden fruits and vegetables) are provided in the following chart in order of toxicity.

1. Strawberries
2. Bell Peppers
3. Spinach
4. Cherries
5. Peaches
6. Cantaloupe
7. Celery
8. Apples
9. Apricots
10. Green Beans
11. Grapes
12. Cucumbers

Food as Medicine

Fatigue is an epidemic, particularly in the United States according to Dr. Victor Zeines holistic dentist and nutritionist. He proposes that fatigue-related ailments should be viewed as "chronic malnutrition." With proper diet, fatigue is simply not an issue. Feeling "awake" and vibrantly alive is an elemental aspect of optimal health. Dr. Ian Brighthope, nutritionist and environmentalist also makes an excellent point that each day you neglect nutrition by eating improperly, you are entering deeper into a state of nutrient deficiency. You cannot make up for poor health by loading up on fruits and veggies every now and again. Nutrition is literally *fuel* for your cells and organs, and you need to feed your body the proper fuel each and every day, not just once in a while. As Dr. Brighthope says, sooner or later you will have to pay for this neglect, and this "payment due," of course, comes in the form of sickness and disease.

Well, since we have come to the understanding that improper nutrition caused the problem (and poor diet is at the heart of nearly ALL disease, from colds and flu's to cancer), it makes sense then that the corrective action needed is *proper* nutrition.

Modern medicine has its place and serves an important function when it comes to major trauma and emergency situations. But many experts will verify that not every problem requires costly, major medical attention. For most diseases, such as type 2 diabetes, heart disease, high blood pressure, chronic fatigue, and autoimmune disorders, just to name a few, there are many natural alternative therapies (including simple dietary changes) that can *be* more effective than conventional medical treatments—not to mention more economical, less harmful and less invasive. ~ Food Matters

WHY Fruits and Vegetables? A Case That Cannot Be Disputed

It is a standard that has been encouraged that we consume 9-13 servings of fruits-and vegetables each day. Your mother may have told you carrots keep your eyes bright as a child, which is still true today. But as an adult, it looks like fruit along with vegetables are just as important for keeping your sight as well as warding off many other forms of sickness and disease. These combined servings of fruit and vegetables may sound like allot to eat each day, but by simply tossing a banana into your morning smoothie or slicing it over your cereal, topping off a cup of Greek yogurt with some berries or having a green salad with a couple of diced pears and snacking on an apple, plum, nectarine or melon, you have reached your daily goal.

The Joy of Healthy Living: The Healing Power of Fruits and Vegetables—a Labor of Love

The background story of how this book came to be is just as fascinating as the book itself. It was originally created to convince my family and friends, to think about proven ways to holistically heal themselves of chronic disease and fatigue. Many of my friends and family have succumb to taking conventional over the counter and prescribed drugs to subdue symptoms of disease such as hypertension, diabetes and cancer. I continued to encourage my friends and family that poor food choice over time were one of the major factors that led to their disease process and healthy food choices ultimately would weave them out of their symptoms into health and vitality. I have felt from time to time like the following quotes written by Ghandi and Arthur Schopenhauer.

First they ignore you, then they laugh at you, then they fight you, then you win.
Mohandas Gandhi

All truth passes through three stages: First, it is ridiculed. Second, it is violently opposed. Third, it is accepted as being self-evident. **Arthur Schopenhauer**

Gandhi and Schopenhauer decisively discussed how we move to the next level but the shifting has to take place within us first. The truth of the healing power of fruits and vegetables is not readily self evident to the masses yet. You and I have much work to do and the most important person I care about right now is YOU. You are reading this book and have the ability to change your health and through your actions teach others to do the same. I once read a wise quote that said "you can not save the person next to you if the plane is going down until you put your oxygen mask on first."

Once you have decided to put on your oxygen mask things get really exciting on the path to living and feeling healthy. When you are actively utilizing "food tools" to heal yourself you are then able to help others, by showing them how to heal themselves and ultimately this is when you help others put on their metaphoric oxygen mask. You can guide others on the path and you can become their oxygen line. Ultimately, you can begin to bring others peace through the knowledge you shall possess.

Once you understand how things work inside you, you will naturally begin to see how they work in others. You will discover how health and wellness work in other people, and see them as insight about and for yourself. To help others, you must help yourself first. If you try to help others initially, you will both remain unconscious to your current plight which will lead to not being able to guide yourself or any one else to the path of natural health and wellness. It takes great courage to help your self before helping another. So let's fit your oxygen mask to help you become conscious. Then you will be in position to help others.

Fruits + Vegetables = Vibrant Health

Of course many of us have grown up knowing that fruits and vegetables are good for the body. But knowing that fruits and vegetables can prevent and alleviate symptoms of chronic disease is usually pushed aside with skepticism. As you read this book begin to reprogram your state of mind on how oranges can help you overcome your common cold and when you consume berries you are enhancing your cardiovascular system. You can heal your body with the right choices in your supermarket basket.

Each animal on earth has their most balanced type of food to eat. In nature, these animals eat their balanced diet to survive and they do not have the health problems we do (unless they are domesticated) and begin living among humans. Now what does that tell you? That we definitely are what we eat. If we were to subscribe to our natural plant based diet, we would unquestionably not have the health issues we have today.

The recipe for your health and overall wellness is simple, with a shift in perception and altering your habits towards an optimal life. You do not need a new and improved drug. You need proper nutrition and the healing power of fruits, vegetables, physical and mental exercise and fresh water. Envision yourself as a baby that you take care of in regards to what it is fed and what it drinks. You may be a bit older than a baby but your health and wellness is just as important now as it was then.

My goal is that over time you will be happy, healthy and fit. I want you to be disease free, drug free, and at your optimal weight enjoying exercise and being healthy mentally and physically. The journey toward self evident truth has now begun.

This book is based on a discussion of Eating Whole Food vs. Ingesting Isolated Vitamins

You will not see many references to isolated vitamins from fruits and vegetables throughout this book even though they are the primary constituents of phytonutrients and antioxidants. The discussion will more so be based on getting the maximum benefit of ingesting the whole food where at times could mean the skin and seeds which usually are discarded but have been found to possess the highest antioxidant levels along with eating fruit and vegetables. The power is in the synergy of the whole fruit vs. isolating it into unsynthesized compounds that in most forms becomes toxic to the body.

Nature intended for us to consume food in its WHOLE form because all the vitamins, minerals, antioxidants and enzymes are together in one package and work synergistically together to bring your body the nutrition that it needs. When you take one part away from the whole, you get "Synthetic", "Isolated" or "Fractionated" pieces of the whole, but it is simply not the same. The other problem is that by taking isolated vitamins, sometimes we are getting "massive" doses of some vitamins, but not enough of others. Over time because we are not receiving the synergistic effect of eating whole foods it can cause health problems.

Phytonutrients, Antioxidants, Flavanoids, Hooray! (Use this section as a resource to the scientific terms used through out this book. These terms clearly show the types of synergistic natural chemicals that sustain health and overall wellness in our bodies.)

Phytonutrients

Many fruits and vegetables contain an abundance of microscopic healing substances known as phytonutrients. These substances are believed to be so powerful that some scientists call them "the vitamins of tomorrow". The discovery of phytonutrients has changed everything we know about fruits and vegetables - one of the most exiting discoveries is that some foods can literally stop chemical changes that can lead to chronic disease.

There are an impressive amount of findings that indicate a promising direction for understanding the molecular mechanisms responsible for the beneficial effects of plant chemicals on human health. **(Please refer to the Documented Resource Section at the end of this book for research references that were used within this book.)**

Anthocyanins

Foods that contain purple-colored pigments called anthocyanins are now being recognized as extra special when it comes to the protection of our blood vessels and our nerve cells. Examples of foods high in anthocyanins include blueberries, bilberries, blackberries, dark cherries, purple carrots, pomegranate, acai, purple sweet potatoes, purple cauliflower, black grapes and beets. Color pigments in berries that are powerful antioxidants of blue, purple, and red have been associated with a lower risk of certain cancers, urinary tract health, memory function, and healthy aging.

Anti-oxidants

Are substances that help neutralize free radicals in your body by stabilizing their chemical structure? They are believed to reduce the physical effects of aging, and possibly prevent disease. The human body produces some antioxidants naturally, while fruits and vegetables provide others

Carotenes

Are you getting enough "orange" foods in your diet? Fruits and vegetables that are naturally orange are usually a good source of carotenoids – natural plant pigments that have a variety of health benefits. Not only are the carotenoids good antioxidants, but they also boost the immune system and help to protect against some chronic diseases. The numbers of carotenoid compounds found in nature are staggering – around six-hundred have currently been described. They are naturally created by plants, – making them an important dietary component. Not surprisingly, unless you eat a fruit and vegetable rich diet, you are probably not getting enough of these healthy compounds.

Orange Veggies

One way to get a healthy dose of carotenoids is to add more orange vegetables to your daily meals. Fall is a perfect time to make pumpkin soup or a pumpkin pie since pumpkin is one of the best sources of carotene around. Other veggies that are rich in carotenoids are sweet potatoes, carrots, and winter squash. With these choices, you can make a "carotene" tasty soup by combining carrots, sweet potatoes, and winter squash.

Green Veggies

It's not just orange vegetables that are rich in carotenoids, some green ones have high quantities too. Good choices are kale, turnip greens, mustard greens, collard greens dandelion greens, swiss chard, watercress, beet greens, and spinach. Let us not forget broccoli which is another green vegetable that has respectable quantities of carotenoids. If you make a salad using carotenoid rich vegetables, use a dressing that has a healthy fat – such as olive oil to balance the release of the carotenoids into your body.

Catechins

Catechins are flavonols that support the antioxidant defense system. Catechins found in cranberries are very similar to those found in green tea which studies show may contribute to cancer prevention.

Dietary Fiber

Found only in plant foods, fiber helps maintain a healthy GI tract, lowers blood cholesterol, reduces heart disease and may prevent certain types of cancers.

Enzymes

There are 2 types of enzymes. They are intra-cellular enzymes and extracellular enzymes. All enzymes are made inside cells. Most of them remain inside the cell to speed up reactions in the cells (intracellular enzymes) while some others are released to work in systems such as the digestive system in stomach. Extracellular enzymes can build up or break down substances. The building up reaction is called "anabolic" while the breaking down reaction is called as "catabolic" reaction.

Gallic Acid

Gallic acid is a potent antioxidant also found in black tea and red wine, shown in tests to inhibit cell proliferation and cell death in prostrate cancer cells.

Lycopene

Lycopene is the pigment that colors your watermelon red, your grapefruit pink and your tomato a deep crimson and it is known to hold potent antioxidant ability. In fact, many studies point to the antioxidant Lycopene as a tool in combating prostate cancer and heart disease, as well as being beneficial in maintaining good prostate health.

Antioxidants can also strengthen the immune system, as well as boost the body's overall level of health. Such potent powers are available to us through foods rich in antioxidants such as Lycopene. Cooking releases Lycopene locked inside plant cells assist the body in absorbing and digesting Lycopene. Good food sources of this powerful antioxidant include ketchup, canned tomatoes, tomato sauce and tomato paste.

Non-digestible Carbohydrates

Non-digestible carbohydrates are a group of carbohydrate substances found in the cell walls of plants and in the tissue between certain plant cells. Pectin, a non digestible carbohydrate is produced by the ripening of fruit and helps the ripe fruit remain firm. Pectins can be made to form gels, and are used in certain natural medicines and cosmetics and in making jellies.

Resveratrol

Resveratrol is one of the phenolic compounds in wine that is thought to reduce serum cholesterol levels when wine is consumed in moderate amounts. Resveratrol is produced in plants during times of environmental stress such as adverse weather or ecological attack. It has been identified in numerous plant species, including mulberries, peanuts, and grapes. Resveratrol is not found in the flesh but in the skin of grapes. Which is why red wines made from grapes stay in contact with the skins much longer than white or rose wines. Resveratrol are associated with reduced risk of heart disease and cancer.

ORAC (Oxygen Radical Absorbance Capacity)

ORAC (Oxygen Radical Absorbance Capacity) values are a measure of the antioxidant activity. Specifically, it measures the degree and length of time it takes to inhibit the action of an oxidizing agent. Antioxidants inhibit oxidation which is known to have a damaging effect on tissues. Studies now suggest that consuming fruits and vegetables with a high

ORAC value may slow the aging process in both body and brain. Antioxidants are shown to work best when combined with the presence of fiber and other plant compounds that enhance the health benefit. For this reason, actually eating fruits and vegetable is a more viable antioxidant option than that of ingesting isolated vitamins.

Phytochemicals

Phytochemicals are naturally occurring antioxidants in plants that add flavor, color pigments and scent, and they are abundant in all types of fruits and vegetables, particularly berries.

The pigments that give berries their rich red to blue, black and purple colors are a type of phytochemical that has been shown to have significant disease-fighting, cell-protecting antioxidant capacity.

Phyto-sterols (plant sterols)

Phytosterols are chemical compounds found in plants and are similar to healthy cholesterol in their structure and function. Plant sterols are soluble fiber, which reduce your low-density lipoprotein (LDL) which is the "bad" cholesterol. Plant sterols were highly prevalent in early human diets that were heavily plant-based. They are currently the focus of cholesterol and cancer cell research.

Quercetin

A flavonol in fruits and vegetables that work as both an anti-carcinogen, an- antioxidant and protects against cancer and heart disease.

Rutin

A bioflavonoid in fruits and vegetables that promotes vascular health. Rutin helps to prevent cell proliferation associated with cancer and has anti-inflammatory and anti-allergenic properties.

Salicylic Acid

The salicylic acid found in cranberries may prove to have the same protective effect against heart disease as aspirin. A handful of red raspberries contain around 5 milligrams of salicylic acid.

Other Overall Benefits of Phytochemicals

Other phytochemicals include detoxifying agents like indoles, isothiocyanates, non- starch polysaccharides or dietary fiber like gums, hemicelluloses, mucilage, pectin, tannins, and alkaloids like caffeine and non-protein amino acids. Dietary fiber increases bulk of the food and helps prevent constipation by decreasing gastro-intestinal transit time. They also bind to toxins in the food and help protect the colon mucus membrane from cancers. In addition, dietary fiber binds to bile salts (produced from cholesterol) and decreases their re-absorption, thus help lower serum LDL cholesterol levels.

When I was first made aware of all of these phytochemicals and antioxidant fighting free radical information, I said to myself that is a mouthful that does not roll off the tongue if you say it more than once. But I began to realize that it was much more than the scientific terms, it was the healing energy of these fruits and vegetables that was derived from the sun, soil and water that were used to produce it. You do not have to say the scientific terms to know that we are all created based on energy and when we get exhausted of that energy, fruits and vegetables are a key to opening the door of our health and wellness potential.

Discover How Fruits Can Heal

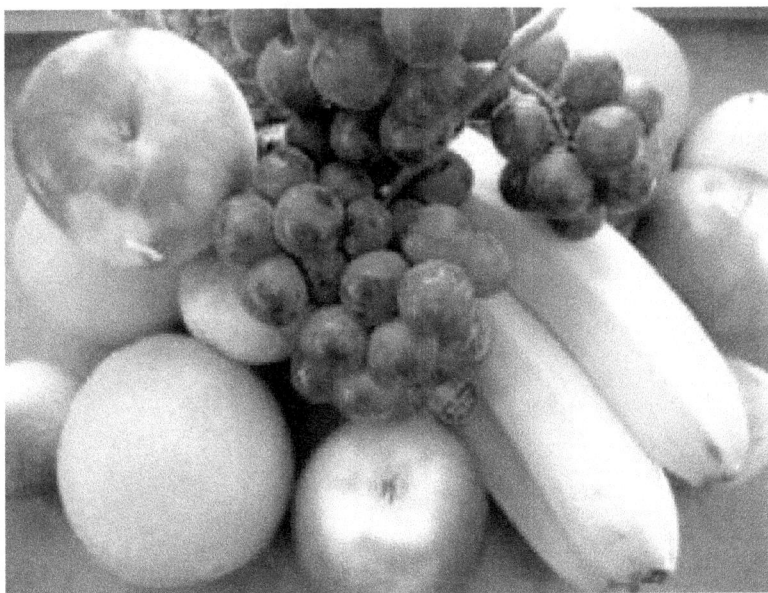

Awesome Apples

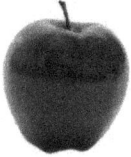

Anyone can count the seeds in an apple, but only God can count the number of apples in a seed." -- Robert H. Schuller

Awesome Apples

Prevent fermentation and bad bacterial growth in intestines

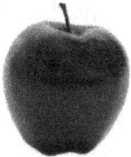

If you have low blood sugar apples stimulate your appetite

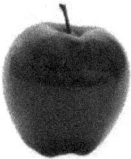

Pectin in apples removes cholesterol, toxic metals and radiation

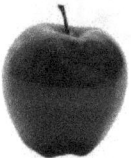

Place apple slices over the eyes for swelling, inflammation-pink eye, and sunburn

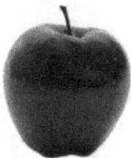

Protects lungs from cigarette smoke

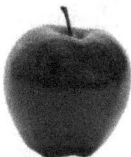

Cleans the gall bladder and softens gallstones

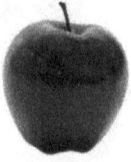

Prevent constipation and blocks diarrhea

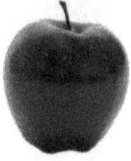

Help reduce cholesterol levels

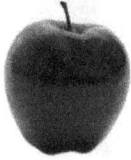

Reduce the risk of coronary heart disease stoke and heart attack in humans.

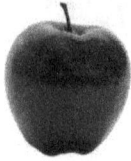

Apples bind carcinogens in the colon that help protect the body from certain types of cancer

Health Benefits of Apples

We all know the saying, "An apple a day keeps the doctor away," but did you know that apples contain substances that have protective and therapeutic values? Known as nutracuticles, they may be just what your body needs for optimum health.

Red apples also contain pectin, which is a soluble fiber that has been found to help lower blood cholesterol levels. Pectin causes the cholesterol in foods to remain in the intestinal tract until it is eliminated from the body. It also binds carcinogens in the colon, which helps protect the body from certain types of cancer.

A group of chemicals in apples protect the brain from the type of damage that triggers neurodegenerative diseases like Alzheimer's and

Parkinson's. It has been found that antioxidants in fresh apples can protect nerve cells from toxicity induced by oxidative stress.

Asthma Help
It has been found that children born to women who eat a lot of apples daily during pregnancy have lower rates of asthma than children whose mothers ate few apples.

Bone Protection
A flavonoid in apples called phloridzin protects post-menopausal women from osteoporosis and may also increase bone density.

Diabetes Management
The pectin in apples supplies natural plant acid to the body which lowers the body's need for insulin and may help in the management of diabetes.

Lower Cholesterol
The pectin in apples lowers LDL "bad" cholesterol.

Lung Cancer Prevention
The flavanoids in apples help lower risk of developing cancer.

Aspiring Apricots

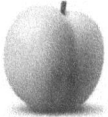

Apricots are gold and delicious. ~ Sarah Peters

Aspiring Apricots

Moistens dry throat.

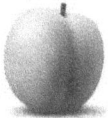

Nourishes blood from anemia

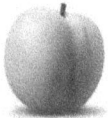

Combats cancer

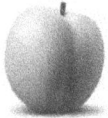

Controls blood pressure

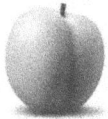

Saves your eyesight

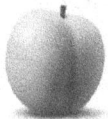

Shields against Alzheimer's

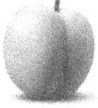

Slows aging process

Health Benefits of Apricots

Apricots are colorful and tasty. They contain several nutrients that promote good health. The fruit, kernels, oil and flowers of the apricot have been used to heal the body for many years. The kernel, which creates oil, has been used for its sedative traits. Apricots have relaxing qualities that give relief to strained muscles and possess soothing properties. They are also useful in the healing of wounds.

Apricots are high in beta-carotene and lycopene, two antioxidant compounds commonly found in orange-red fruits and vegetables that promote heart health and prevent several types of cancers. Beta-carotene and lycopene also protect LDL cholesterol from oxidation, reducing the risk of developing atherosclerosis and several cardiovascular diseases.

Apricots are high in antioxidants that promote the blood supply to the eyes and cause macular degeneration.

Apricots are also a good source of fiber, which have several health benefits especially related to the health of the digestive tract which prevents constipation and cancer-promoting conditions due to lack of expelling toxicity.

Anemia

Apricots are high in iron and can be used to alleviate anemia. The amount of copper in the fruit makes iron available to the body. Consistent use of apricots could also increase the production of hemoglobin in our body.

Constipation

The fruit of the apricot can be used as a gentle laxative and is beneficial in the treatment of constipation. The indigestible fiber of apricots acts as roughage which helps bowel movement. Pectin in apricots absorb and retains water which increases the bulk of feces and stimulates smooth bowel movement.

Fevers

Fresh juice of apricots, mixed with honey, is a cooling drink during fevers. It eliminates the waste products from the body. It tones up the eyes, stomach, liver, heart and nerves by supplying nutrients that are depleted due to fever.

Indigestion

Apricots have an alkaline reaction in the system. They aid the digestion, if consumed before a meal. Marmalade, made from organically grown apricots, is also valuable in the treatment of nervous indigestion.

Skin Diseases

Fresh juice of apricot leaves is useful in treating skin diseases. It can be applied with beneficial results in scabies, eczema, sun-burn and itching of the skin due to cold exposure.

Bodacious Bananas

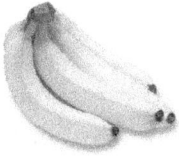

Even without drumbeats, banana leaves dance. ~ African Proverb

Bodacious Bananas

Treats dry cough

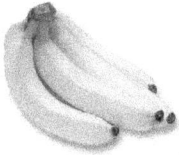

Alleviates diarrhea, hemorrhoids, and colitis

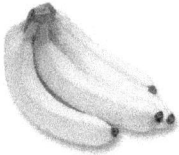

Lowers blood pressure

*Due to blood pressure reduction effects use with caution on children who are cold, inactive or frail.

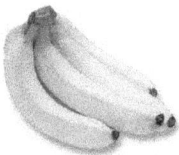

Protects your heart

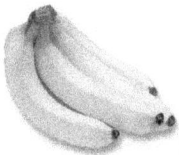

Strengthens your bones

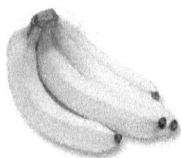

Heightens serotonin levels that make you feel happy

Natural Health Benefits of Bananas

Bananas promote serotonin in the body. Serotonin is used for treating depression so eating a banana can elevate your mood positively, help you relax and feel happier. A banana gives instant, sustained boost of energy. But energy is not the only way a banana can help us keep fit. It can also help to overcome or prevent a substantial number of illnesses and conditions, making it a must to add to our daily diet.

Anemia
High in iron, bananas can stimulate the production of hemoglobin in the blood and helps in cases of anemia.

Blood Pressure
Bananas are extremely high in potassium yet low in salt, making it perfect to beat high blood pressure.

Brain Power
It has been shown that the potassium-packed fruit can assist learning by making students more alert.

Constipation
High in fiber, including bananas in the diet can help restore normal bowel action.

Heartburn
Bananas have a natural antacid effect in the body, so if you suffer from heartburn, try eating a banana for soothing relief.

Morning Sickness

Snacking on bananas between meals help to keep blood sugar levels up and avoid morning sickness.

Mosquito bites

Before reaching for the insect bite cream, try rubbing the affected area with the inside of a banana skin. Many people find it amazingly successful at reducing swelling and irritation.

Nerves

Bananas are high in phytonutrients that help calm the nervous system.

PMS

Forget the pills - eat a banana. The phytonutrients in bananas regulate blood glucose levels, which can affect your mood.

Temperature control

Many other cultures see bananas as a "cooling" fruit that can lower both the physical and emotional temperature of expectant mothers.

Ulcers:

The banana is used as the dietary food against intestinal disorders because of its soft texture and smoothness. It also neutralizes over-acidity and reduces irritation by coating the lining of the stomach.

Over coming Smoking & Tobacco Use:

Bananas can also help people trying to give up smoking. The B6, B12 they contain, as well as the potassium and magnesium found in them, help the body recover from the effects of nicotine withdrawal.

Strokes:

Eating more bananas as part of a regular diet can cut the risk of death by strokes because they enhance cardiovascular system activity.

Warts:

The healing properties of bananas promote healthy skin growth. If you want to kill off a wart, take a piece of banana skin and place it on the wart, with the yellow side of the banana skin facing out. Keep the banana skin in place while changing it with fresh banana skin until your skin is healed.

Bountiful Blackberry

Blackberries are like dark pearls that you can eat. ~ Sarah McPeters

Bountiful Blackberry

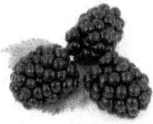

Lowers risk of cancer

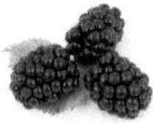

Supports healthy urinary tract

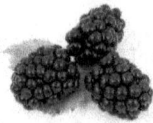

Supports memory function

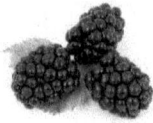

Declines inflammation

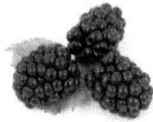

Treats diarrhea

Bountiful Blackberries

Blackberry fruit contains vast amounts of anthocyanocides, which are found in the pigment that gives the berries their color. Anthocyanocides are powerful antioxidants that help to reverse cell damage caused by free radicals, and are reported to be instrumental in preventing heart disease, cancer and strokes.

Blackberry leaves are used in making blackberry tea and can be used in treating non-specific acute diarrhea, as well as inflammation of the mouth and throat. It is also reported to be helpful in reducing blood sugar levels.

To prepare blackberry tea add 1 heaping tablespoon of dried blackberry tea leaves per cup of boiling water, cover, and steep 10 minutes. Strain and add honey or brown sugar to taste. You can combine equal amounts of dried mint and dried blackberry tea leaves as a nourishing combination.

Blackberries (also known as black raspberries) reduce the risk of esophageal cancer by reducing the oxidative stress that result from a precancerous condition usually caused by gastro-esophageal reflux disease.

High in Antioxidants
Blackberries are one of the top ten foods containing antioxidants.

Helps Prevent Cancer
Blackberries are packed with polyphenols helping to prevent cancer and heart disease. Blackberries have been found to protect against esophageal cancer, a cancer caused by gastric reflux disease. Blackberries have been shown to protect against other types of cancers. They contain phytoestrogens (plant estrogens), a compound believed to play a vital role in preventing breast and cervical cancer.

Helps Memory Retention
Blackberries are filled with anthocyanins, which are antioxidants that

give blackberries their deep purple color which help in memory retention and reduce the risk of hypertension.

Strengthens Blood Vessels
Blackberries are said to strengthen blood vessels, help fight heart disease and help improve eyesight.

Strengthens Intestinal Tract
The high tannin content of blackberries help tighten tissue, relieve intestinal inflammation, and help reduce hemorrhoids and stomach disorders.

High in Fiber
The high fiber content of blackberries help reduce risk of intestinal disease and the risk of developing diabetes.

Beautiful Black Currant

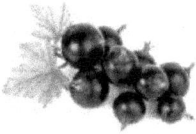

Black currants in a wine press are sweeter than honey. ~ Wine of Its Time

Beautiful Black Currant

Treats cardiovascular disease

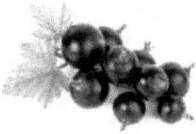

Reduces hypertension

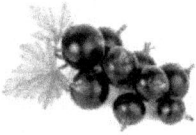

Detoxifies the blood

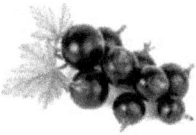

Reduces cholesterol

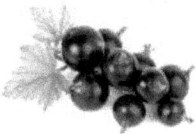

Useful against rheumatoid arthritis

Black Currant Health Benefits

The fruits, leaves and buds of the black currant have multiple effects in treating and preventing various diseases. Black currant is used in treating cardiovascular diseases, preventing cardiac insufficiency and vascular accidents, it increases the resistance of fragile sanguine capillaries, reduces arterial hypertension. Also, it intensifies weak peripheral circulation caused by menopause; it also cleans the blood of toxins, wastes and cholesterol.

When you add black currant to the diet it is useful against rheumatism, arthritis and gout. The plant stimulates digestion and functioning of the liver, pancreas, spleen and kidneys.

Being an astringent, this fruit is useful against diarrhea and dysentery. Black currants are also useful against tiredness and overwork. Black currant is recommended as a systemic anti-inflammatory agent with actions similar to those of natural cortisone, in acute and chronic allergies such as bronchial asthma, allergic rhinitis, and diabetic retinopathy. In external use, the mixtures from black currant fruits are used for treating abscess, dermatitis, eczemas and insect stings.

High Antioxidant Level and Cancer Reduction
Black currant is high in the antioxidant named anthocyanin, which protects against liver cancer.

Fortifies the body
Black currant fortifies the body including blood vessels and muscles.

Promotes Cardiovascular Wellness
Black currant helps normalize blood pressure, heart function, muscle and nerve activity.

Brainy Blueberries

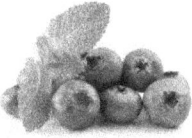

If all the blueberries grown in North America in one year were spread out in a single layer, they would cover a four-lane highway that stretched from New York to Chicago. ~(The Great Food Almanac)

Brainy Blueberries

Blueberries have been shown to shrink cancerous tumors and prevent the development and growth of cancer cells

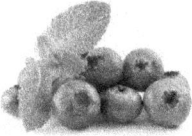

Blueberries can slow down and even reverse age-related memory loss

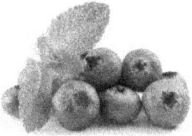

Blueberries can help improve physical coordination and balance at an advanced age

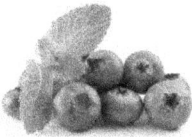

Blueberries reduce cholesterol levels

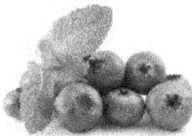

Blueberries prevent urinary tract infections

Health Benefits of Blueberries

Besides these astounding health benefits, blueberries are also nutritional powerhouses. They are low in calories and high in fiber.

They rank among the top providers of antioxidants which are essential to nutritional health. Antioxidants like anthocyanin, among other important micronutrients, boost the immune system and help to prevent infection.

In addition to its rich nutritional qualities, blueberries have the ability to neutralize "free radicals," which are unstable molecules that can cause many diseases and accelerate the aging process. This is mainly due to the concentrated presence of anthocyanin, the pigment that gives berries their dark bluish color.

Berries should always be purchased organic because of the permeable nature of the skin of berries which are susceptible to pesticides that are used to increase their yield.

Lower Cholesterol Levels
A diet rich in blueberries lowers blood cholesterol levels while improving glucose control and insulin sensitivity which helps lower the risk of subsequent heart disease and diabetes.

Immunity Builder
Blueberries have the highest antioxidant capacity of all fresh fruit: Blue berries, are rich in anti oxidants like anthocyanin that are an effective immune builder and anti-bacterial. With a strong immune system you are less prone to get colds, fever, pox and other such viral and bacterial communicable diseases.

Promotes Urinary Tract Health
Blueberries inhibit the growth of bad bacteria. The also cleanse away bacteria along the urinary tract, thereby preventing infection.

Preserve Vision
Blueberry has been found in clinical studies to slow down visual loss. They prevent or delay all age related ocular problems like macular degeneration, cataract, myopia and hypermetropia, dryness and

infections, particularly those pertaining to the retina, due to their anti-oxidant properties.

Brain Health:
Blueberries have been found to promote healthy brain-cell growth. They have also been found to restore health of the central nervous system. These berries can also be used to treat serious problems like Alzheimer's disease to a great extent. They even heal damaged brain cells and neuron tissue that keep your memory sharp for a long time.

Promotes a Healthy Heart
The high fiber content, those brilliant anti-oxidants and the ability to dissolve the 'bad cholesterol' make the blue berry an ideal dietary supplement to cure many heart diseases. It also strengthens the cardiac muscles.

Healthy Digestion:
Fiber in blueberries keep away constipation and promote ease of digestion.

Positive Mood Enhancer
Blueberries keep you fresh, active, fit, sharp, and in a good mood. They are good anti-depressants. Remember, the deeper the color of the blue berries, the more they are rich in anti oxidants and other medicinal values.

Courageous Cantaloupe

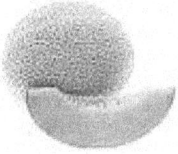

"How should melon be eaten? Not with a spoon, as is usual in restaurants.....The back of the spoon anaesthetizes the taste buds! In this way, it loses half of its flavor. Melon should be eaten with a fork."~ **From article 'Propos de table' by J. De Coquet in June 1982 'Figaro'**

Courageous Cantaloupe

Saves eyesight

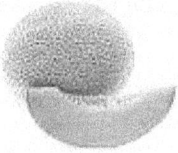

Controls blood pressure

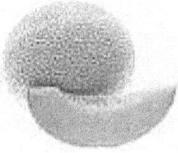

Lowers cholesterol

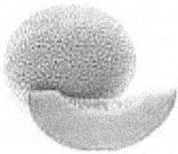

Combats cancer

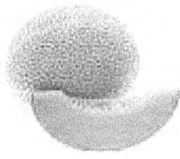

Supports your immune system

Cantaloupe Health Benefits

Cantaloupe with its refreshingly rich flavor and aroma is one of the most popular forms of melon. Cantaloupe has antioxidants that help us fight heart disease, high blood pressure, diabetes, cancer, and aging. Cantaloupe is also a good source of dietary fiber.

It is an exceptional fruit for supporting energy production through good carbohydrate metabolism and blood sugar stability. Cantaloupe is fat and cholesterol free, and is a great source of foliate.

Folate is necessary for the production and maintenance of new cells, and is especially important during periods of rapid cell division and growth such as infancy and pregnancy.

Promotes Healthy Skin

High doses of vitamin A supplements can be toxic, but getting the nutrient from natural sources such as the cantaloupe is perfectly safe and will even help minimize acne and wrinkles.

Helps Combat Infection

A delicious way to prepare cantaloupe is to make it into a smoothie, a perfect drink for kids and grownups alike to help strengthen the immune system and thus fight off viruses which can cause sickness.

Prevents Urinary Tract Infection

In addition to its high water content which helps flush out the bacteria from your system cantaloupe also works to increase the acidity level of urine, decreasing the harmful microbes that may be present in the urinary tract.

Promotes Fast Healing of Wounds
Add cantaloupe in salads or eat as is to help form collagen, the protein which makes skin and scar tissue.

Helps Lower Blood Pressure Levels
Cantaloupe helps in fighting hypertension by slowing down the effects of sodium in the body.

Promotes Fertility
Planning to have a baby? Don't forget to include one of the richest source of folate in your diet—the cantaloupe. Folate, also called folic acid, is widely known for its importance in pregnancy especially in its vital role in reducing the risk of nervous system problems in newborn babies.

Cherished Cherry

"Most of those who make collections of verse or epigram are like men eating cherries or oysters: they choose out the best at first, and end by eating all." ~Chamfort

Cherished Cherry

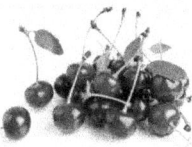
Alleviates Gout, Arthritis, Rheumatism

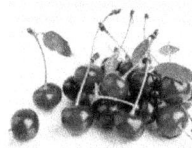
Helps the excretion of body acids

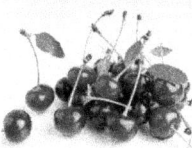
Helps with anemia and weak muscles

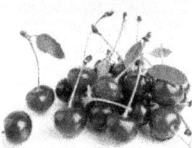
Protects your heart

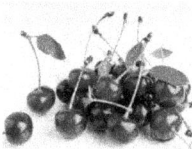
Combats cancer

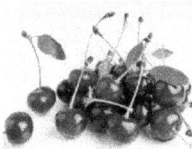
Alleviates insomnia

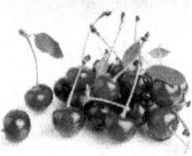

Slows the aging process

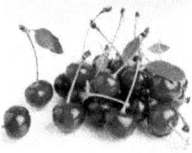

Shields against Alzheimers

Health Benefits of Cherries

Tasty cherries have been shown to decrease the incidence of cancer including those of the breasts, lungs, stomach, liver, and skin. Cherries have a huge beneficial effect when eaten raw as a part of a well – balanced diet. Cherries play an important role in helping the body ward off a number of diseases.

For a long time, it has been known that cherries have been used to treat painful gout conditions. Drinking two glasses a day of cherry juice diluted with equal amount of water daily helps to elevate painful condition of gout.

Cooking destroys some of the nutrients in cherries so it is best to eat them raw to reap their full nutritional benefit.

Reduction of Heart Disease and Cancer

Cherries are packed with antioxidants called anthocyanins which aid in the reduction of heart disease and cancer.

Promotes Restful Sleep

Cherries are one of the few food sources that contain melatonin, an antioxidant that helps regulate heart rhythms and the body's sleep cycles.

Brain Food

Cherries are referred to as "brain food", aiding the brain reception levels and overall health in the prevention of memory loss.

Promotes Digestive Health

Cherries are a good source of fiber which is important for digestive health.

Reduce Inflammation

Because cherries contain anthocyanins, they can reduce inflammation and symptoms of arthritis and gout.

Caring Coconut

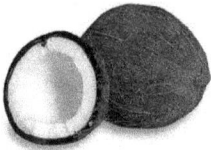

There is sweet water inside a tender coconut. Who poured the water inside the coconut? Was it the work of any man? No. Only God can do such a thing. ~ Hawaiian   Proverb

Caring Coconut

Prevents goiter

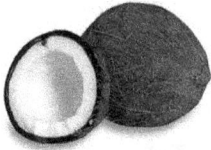

Good for building muscles

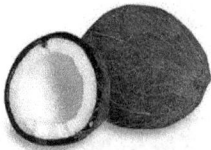

Creates consistent bowel movement

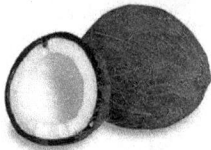

Relieves stomach ulcers

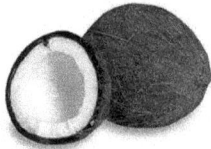

Supports healthy kidneys

Coconut Oil Health Benefits

Coconut is a tropical fruit that is rich in protein. The meat of the coconut is good for destroying intestinal parasites that we get from eating infected food. Coconut water is beneficial for kidney and urinary bladder problems.

Coconut oil is rich in lauric acid, which is known for being anti-viral, antibacterial and anti-fungal. Coconut oil has been used by thyroid sufferers to increase body metabolism, and to lose weight. Virgin coconut oil is used for making natural soaps and other health products, as it is one of the healthiest applications one can put on their skin.

At one time coconut oil received negative press in the US because of its high level of saturated fat. However, modern research has shown that not all saturated fats are alike and that the fatty acids in coconut oil, the medium chain triglycerides, do not raise serum cholesterol or contribute to heart disease, but are in fact very healthy. Also, some negative studies done on coconut oil in the past were done on hydrogenated coconut oil, which has been altered from its original form. Other studies have clearly shown that traditional Asian cultures that eat significant amounts of coconut in their diet do not suffer from modern diseases seen in western cultures that promote a low-fat diet.

As a "functional food," coconut oil is now being recognized by the medical community as a powerful tool against immune diseases. Several studies have been done on its effectiveness, and much research is currently being done on the incredible nutritional value of pure coconut oil.

Eradicates Bacteria, Viruses and Parasites

Supports and aids immune system function. Coconut promotes eradication of viruses that cause influenza, herpes, measles, hepatitis C, and SARS, Coconut also: promotes eradication of bacteria that cause ulcers, throat infections, urinary tract infections, gum disease and cavities, pneumonia, and gonorrhea.

Coconut promotes eradication of fungi and yeasts that cause candidacies, ringworm, athlete's foot, thrush, diaper rash, and other infections. It also rids the body of tapeworms, lice and other parasites.

Relieves Symptoms of Diabetes
Coconut improves insulin secretion and utilization of blood glucose. Relieves stress on pancreas and enzyme systems of the body.

Promotes Strong Teeth and Bones
Improves calcium absorption and supports the development of strong bones and teeth. Helps protect against osteoporosis. Helps prevent periodontal disease and tooth decay.

Reduces Inflammation and Cancer
Coconut reduces inflammation. Helps protect the body from breast, colon, and other cancers.

Functions as a protective antioxidant.
Helps to protect the body from harmful free radicals that promote premature aging and degenerative disease. Helps relieve symptoms associated with chronic fatigue syndrome.

Prevents Goiter
Coconut prevents simple goiter (enlarged non-toxic thyroid) because of its organic iodine content.

Helps Build Muscle
Coconut is recommended for building up the body muscles of thin and emaciated individuals.

Promotes Digestion and Detoxification

Relives constipation for any build-up of gas in the stomach and intestinal tract. Coconut water is good for kidney and urinary bladder problems. It helps relieve symptoms associated with gallbladder disease. Coconut relieves symptoms associated with Crohn's disease, ulcerative colitis, and stomach ulcers. It improves digestion and bowel function.

Coconut relieves pain and irritation caused by hemorrhoids and dissolves kidney stones. Coconut helps prevent liver disease.

Promotes Healthy Skin and Tissue Growth

Coconut milk has been found to help cases of sore throat as well as relieving stomach ulcers.

Coconut oil has been found to heal cuts, scratches, burns and sunburns. The oil has also been recommended for facial massage and is reported to be good as a wrinkle remover. Coconut oil is also good for the scalp and hair. Coconut oil helps control dandruff.

Coconut oil applied topically helps to form a chemical barrier on the skin to ward of infection. It reduces symptoms associated with psoriasis, eczema, and dermatitis. It supports the natural chemical balance of the skin. Coconut oil softens the skin and helps relieve dryness and flaking. It prevents wrinkles, sagging skin, and age spots.

Charming Cranberry

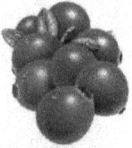

"There are four unbroken rules when it comes to Thanksgiving: there must be turkey and dressing, cranberries, mashed potatoes, and pumpkin pie."~ John Hadamuscin 'John Hadamuscin's Down Home' (1993)

Charming Cranberry

Protection against urinary tract infections

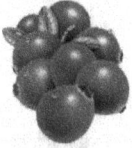

Antinflamitory benefits

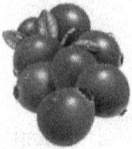

Supports healthy kidney

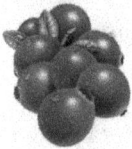

Supports healthy immune system

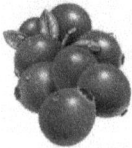

Anti-cancer benefits

Health Benefits of Cranberries

Among the fruits and vegetables richest in health-promoting

antioxidants, cranberries rank high up there at the top of the list. For the cardiovascular system and for many parts of the digestive tract (including the mouth and gums, stomach, and colon) cranberry has been shown to provide important anti-inflammatory benefits. The phytonutrients in cranberry are especially effective in lowering our risk of unwanted inflammation.

Healthy Urinary Tract
Cranberries have long been valued for their ability to help prevent and treat urinary tract infections.

Digestive Tract Benefits
Now, recent studies suggest that this native American berry may also promote gastrointestinal health.

Recent research has also shown that cranberry may be able to help optimize the balance of bacteria.

Promotes Good Cholesterol
Cranberries help lower LDL and raise HDL (good) cholesterol which aids in recovery from stroke,

Prevent Inflammation and Cancer
Since cranberry is loaded with antioxidant and anti-inflammatory nutrients. Chronic excessive oxidative stress (from lack of sufficient antioxidant support) and chronic excessive inflammation (from lack of sufficient anti-inflammatory compounds) are two key risk factors promoting increased likelihood of cancer. With its unique array of antioxidant and anti-inflammatory nutrients, cranberry seems ideally positioned to help us lower our risk of cancer development.

Fresh vs. Frozen Cranberries

When cranberries' short fresh season is past, rely on unsweetened cranberry juice made from whole berries and dried or frozen cranberries to help make every day throughout the year a holiday from disease.

Helps Healthy Skin and Tissue Growth

Cranberries can be used as a poultice for wounds since not only do their astringent tannins contract tissues and help stop bleeding, but we now also know that compounds in cranberries have antibiotic effects.

When you add up the health-related benefits of cranberry for our mouth and gums cranberries also lead to decreased risk of periodontal disease.

Beneficial Deep Red Color

Cranberries that have a deeper red color are more highly concentrated with phytonutrients. Dark red cranberries have been found to have the highest concentration of anthocyanins.

Healthiest Way of Preparing Cranberries

Cranberries retain their maximum amount of nutrients and their maximum taste when they are enjoyed fresh and not prepared in a cooked recipe. That is because their nutrients, antioxidants, and enzymes—are unable to withstand the temperature (350°F/175°C) used in baking.

Favorite Fig

"Fig Newton: The force required to accelerate a fig 39.37 inches per second."
~Johnny Hart, cartoonist (1931-2007)

Favorite Fig

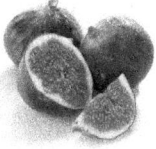

Detox for skin of ulcerations and boils

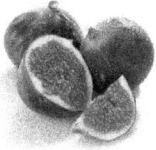

Alleviates dry cough

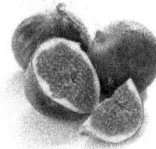

Alleviates asthma symptoms

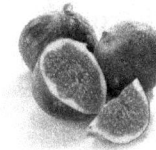

Alleviates sore throat

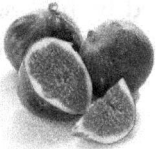

High mucin (protein that makes natural mucous) which makes figs a great laxative

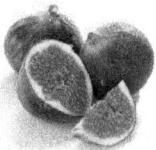

Treats dysentery (inflammatory disorder of the intestine) and hemorrhoids

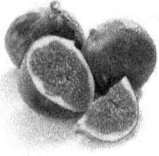

Very alkaline, balances diets high in meats

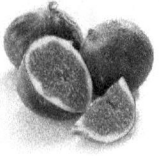

Milk from unripe fig applied twice a day helps to alleviate warts

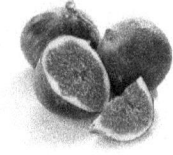

Fresh fig rubbed in gums helps toothache

Fig Health Benefits

You probably do not think about the leaves of the fig tree as one of fig's edible parts. But in some cultures, fig leaves are a common part of the menu, and for good reason. The leaves of the fig have repeatedly been shown to have anti-diabetic properties and can actually reduce the amount of insulin needed by people with diabetes who require insulin injections. To take advantage, you can add fig-leaf extract with breakfast, first thing in the morning, or boil the fig leaves in some fresh filtered water and drink it as tea.

Bone Density Promoter

Figs' counteract the increased urinary calcium loss caused by high-salt diets thus helping to further prevent bones from thinning out at a fast rate.

Cardiovascular Effects

Fig leaves have been shown to lower levels of fat in cells.

Lowers Blood Pressure

Figs are rich in potassium, a mineral that helps to control blood pressure. Studies have shown that people who consume foods with more potassium have lower blood pressure than those who consume less.

Prevents constipation:
Figs create a laxative effect, when consumed daily. Fresh figs and dried ones are equally effective.

Protects Against Postmenopausal Breast Cancer:
It has been found that consuming figs that are high in fiber reduce the risk of breast cancer.

Prevents Heart Disease
Studies have shown that fig leaves can lower fat in the blood stream, thus preventing cardiovascular diseases.

Promotes Bone Density
Figs are rich in calcium, a mineral that strengthens bone density and promote bones. Figs are a good source of potassium which also prevents the loss of urinary calcium caused by high salt diets and leads to bone-thinning.

Great Grapefruit

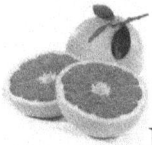

"The taste seemed to come in two parts - a sort of awakening sharpness followed quickly by a wash of sweetness; and each of those little globules (which were about the size of tadpoles) seemed to burst separately in my mouth. That was the grapefruit of my dreams, I don't mind telling you." Julian Barnes, 'A History of the World in 10 1/2 Chapters' (1989)

Great Grapefruit

Protects against heart attack

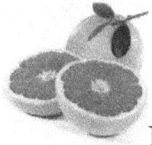

Promotes weight loss

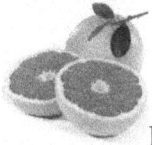

Helps stop strokes

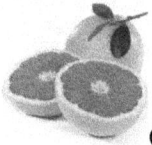

Combats cancer

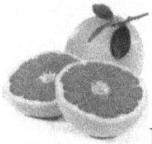

Kills bacteria

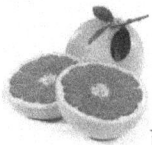

Fights fungus

Grapefruit Health Benefits

It has been found that consumption of grapefruit is associated with a reduced risk heart disease, stroke and cancer. The rich pink and red colors of grapefruit are due to lycopene, a carotenoid phytonutrient. Lycopene appears to have anti-tumor activity. Among the common dietary carotenoids, lycopene has the highest capacity to help fight oxygen free radicals, which are compounds that can damage cells. A similar inverse association was found between the men's consumption of lycopene-rich fruits such as pink grapefruit. Men who most frequently enjoyed these foods were less likely to have prostate cancer compared to those consuming the least lycopene-rich foods.

Phytonutrient Rich Grapefruit

Phytonutrients in grapefruit called limonoids inhibit tumor formation by promoting the creation of a detoxifying enzyme. This enzyme sparks a reaction in the liver that helps to make toxic compounds more water soluble for excretion from the body. Pulp of citrus fruits like grapefruit contain compounds that may help prevent breast cancer.

Grapefruit Lowers Cholesterol

Grapefruit contains pectin, a form of soluble fiber that has been shown in animal studies to slow down the progression of atherosclerosis. Both blond and red grapefruit can reduce blood levels of LDL "bad" cholesterol, and red grapefruit lowers triglycerides as well.

Both red and blond grapefruits positively influence cholesterol levels, but red grapefruit are more than twice as effective, especially in lowering triglycerides. In addition, both grapefruits significantly improve blood levels of protective antioxidants.

Grapefruit Protects against Cancer and Repairs DNA

Grapefruit, helps repair damaged DNA in human prostate cancer cells. The risk of prostate cancer, the most commonly diagnosed cancer in men in the U.S, increases with age since the older we become, the more times our cells have divided and the greater the chance for DNA mutations to occur. DNA repair is one of the body's primary defense mechanisms against the development of cancer since it removes potentially cancer-causing mutations in cells.

Unlike many other cancers, prostate cancer is slow growing initially and often remains undetectable for a long time. Enjoying grapefruit regularly may be one way to prevent its progression by promoting the repair of damaged DNA in prostate cells, thus preventing them from becoming cancerous.

Gracious Grapes

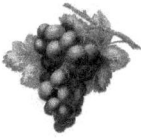

I've been into the habit of freezing white grapes and using them as a snack. Instead of eating peanuts or popcorn or something like that or pretzels, I just eat the white grapes. ~ Mike Ditka

Gracious Grapes

Saves eyesight

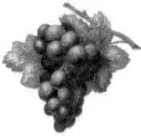

Conquers kidney stones

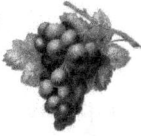

Combats cancer

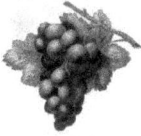

Enhances blood flow

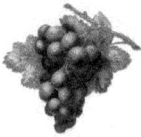

Protects your heart

Health Benefits of Grapes

Grapes have an immense number of health-supportive phytonutrients. Grapes have been shown to provide many of our body systems with predictable benefits. Areas of benefit in grape research include the cardiovascular system, respiratory system, immune system, inflammatory system, blood sugar regulating system, and nervous system. Another area of special benefit is cancer prevention, with risk of breast, prostate, and colon cancer showing grape anti-cancer benefits.

Grapes and Better Blood Sugar Balance

Low glycemic index values of grapes are a good indicator of this fruit's blood sugar benefits. Better blood sugar balance, better insulin regulation, and increased insulin sensitivity has been connected with intake of grape juices, grape extracts, and individual phytonutrients found in grapes.

Grapes and Anti-aging

Several grape phytonutrients are now believed to play a role in anti-aging due to its high amount of resveratrol.

Antioxidant Benefits of Grapes Skin and Seeds

It is important to note that the seed and the skin of grapes contain the richest concentration of antioxidants. It is rare to find a higher concentration of an antioxidant in the fleshy part of the grape than is present in the seed or skin. The best way to get the most concentrated form of antioxidants is to eat the grape: skin, seeds and flesh.

Grapes Improve Metabolism

Grapes are known to treat metabolism disorders: in the liver, kidney and lungs as well as cardiovascular problems. Grapes improve metabolism and have diuretic and anti inflammation effects.

Grapes help with nervous exhaustion, hypertension, high blood pressure, bronchitis and gout. Eating grapes strengthens your body when you need to recover from anemia, gastritis, metabolism disorder, chronic insomnia and constipation.

Raisins Promote Healthy Tissue Growth

You should eat raisins, if you have strained throat tissue due to coughing, have angina, ulcers in your mouth, bladder disorders and hemorrhoids.

Anti-Inflammatory Benefits

Along with their strong antioxidant support, grapes provide us with equally strong anti-inflammatory benefits.

Cardiovascular Benefits

The list of cardio benefits provided by grapes and grape components is perhaps the most extensive. In regards to benefitting the cardiovascular system grapes provide better blood pressure regulation, including blood pressure reduction. Other cardiovascular benefits:

- better total cholesterol regulation and reduction if high

- reduced LDL cholesterol levels

- reduced LDL oxidation

- reduced levels of reactive oxygen molecules in the blood

- reduced likelihood of cell adhesion to the blood vessel walls

- positive flow of platelet cells

- better inflammatory regulation in the blood

Anti-Cancer Benefits

The antioxidant and anti-inflammatory properties of grapes make them a natural for protection against cancer because chronic oxidative stress and chronic inflammation can be key factors in the development of cancer.

Skin vs. Skinless Grapes

While some recipes call for peeled grapes, see if you can include the skin due to grape skin containing the fruit's vital nutrients.

Luscious Lemons

"When fate hands you a lemon, make lemonade." ~ Dale Carnegie

Luscious Lemons

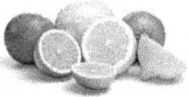

Combats cancer

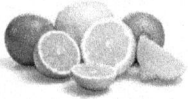

Protects your heart

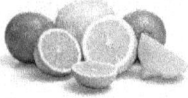

Controls blood pressure

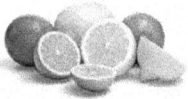

Smoothes skin

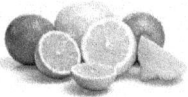

Stops scurvy

Luscious Lemons/Limes

Lemons/Limes Health Benefits

Both of these high antioxidant citrus fruits carry out many of the same beneficial properties in the body so they have been grouped and used interchangeably in this section that focuses on their health benefits. Lemons and limes offer unique phytonutrients. Lemons and limes contain flavanoids that have antioxidant and anti-cancer properties. While these flavonoids have been shown to stop cell division (duplication) in many cancer cell lines, they are perhaps most interesting for their antibiotic effects.

Lemons/Limes helping Cells Choose Life

One of the greatest healing properties of lemons and limes are demonstrated through their ability to alter the choice progression of our cells. This is shown through our cell cycles. In a cell cycle, cells make the decision as to whether to divide and thrive through duplication or die. This is most apparent in cell duplication in a healthy immune system where the nutrients of lemons and limes have been consistently utilized to promoting thriving cells.

Lemons /Limes Support Optimal Health

Lemons and limes have been shown to help fight cancers of the mouth, skin, lung, breast, stomach and colon. Lemons and limes bioavailability and persistence have been shown to be potent anti-carcinogens that prevent cancerous cells from growing.

Lemons/Limes as a Salt Substitute

Lemons and limes are a great substitute if you are watching your salt intake, serve lemon wedges with meals as their tartness amplifies the taste of the food it is added to.

Lemon Alleviating Blood Pressure

The phytonutrients in lemons benefit people with high blood pressure. Lemons control dizziness, nausea and high blood pressure, which consequently reduce the risk of heart disease.

Lemons/Limes Promote Digestion

Lemons/Limes alleviate heartburn, nausea, bloating, belching and parasites. Lemons take care of constipation problems, by clearing the bowels. Lemons are helpful for the liver because they produce more bile, which in turn speeds up the process of digestion.

Lemons/Limes Creates Vibrant Skin

Lemons/Limes have the ability to remove blemishes of the skin such as blackheads and wrinkles. Ingesting lemons over time removes scars and dark patches on the skin.

Lemons/Limes Promotes Healthy Teeth and Gums

Lemons/Limes reduce toothache and cures wounds when massaged on gums. Lemons can also be used to freshen your breath.

Lemons/Limes Clears the Throat

Lemons/Limes fight infection in the throat. The best remedy for sore throat is to gargle with fresh lemon juice mixed in warm water.

Lemons /Limes for Respiratory Problems

Lemons/Limes clear chest congestion by loosening congestion in the respiratory track.

Lemons /Limes Expels Toxins

Lemons/Limes are a natural diuretic. In addition the detoxifying property of lemon juice can help the body to flush out toxins from your system.

Magnificent Mangoes

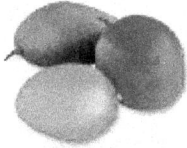

Mangoes are the jewels of sweet trees. ~D. Francis

Magnificent Mangoes

Combats cancer

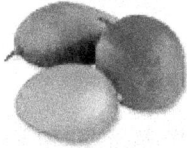

Boost memory

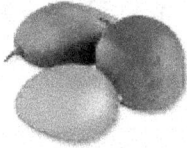

Regulates thyroid

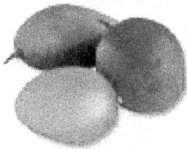

Aids digestion

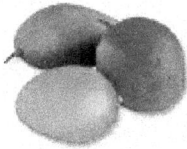

Shields against Alzheimer's

Mango Health Benefits

The phytonutrients in mangoes are durable in preventing disease processes from progressing. Mango is also high in a soluble dietary fiber. The fiber of mangoes and potent antioxidants lower the risk of free radical damage and reduces risk of cancer.

Improves Digestion

Mangoes are beneficial for people suffering from acidity because mangoes alkalinizes the body and its enzymes help to relieve indigestion problems.

Lowers Cholesterol

High level of soluble dietary fiber in mangoes help lower cholesterol levels specifically (LDL) Cholesterol.

Improves Concentration and Memory Power

Mangoes are useful to children who lack concentration in studies as it contains phytonutrients which boost memory and keep cells active.

For Treating Acne

Mango helps in clearing clogged pores that cause acne. Just slice the mango into thin pieces and keep it on your face for 10 to 15 minutes then take a bath and wash your face. Use warm water for washing your face and cleansing your pores.

High in Iron

Mangoes are rich in iron. People who suffer from anemia can regularly take mango along with their daily meals and/or during snacking to lessen occurrences of anemia.

Nice Nectarine

Talking of pleasure, this moment I was writing with one hand, and with the other holding to my mouth a nectarine -- how good how fine. It went down all pulpy, slushy, oozy, its entire delicious embodiment melted down my throat like a large, beautified strawberry." John Keats (1795-1821)

Nice Nectarine

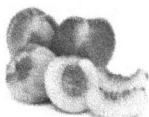

Helps boost the immune system

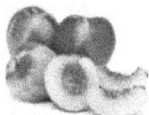

Promotes healthy skin

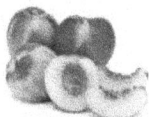

Helps control blood pressure

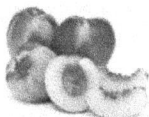

Anti-cancer promotion

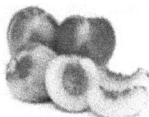

Alleviates constipation

Health Benefits of Nectarines
Nectarines are packed with numerous health promoting anti-oxidants and plant nutrients. These antioxidants are a vital force in creating

healthy synthesis within connective tissue. Nectarines help the body to develop resistance against infection and free radical damage.

Nectarines Help Create Optimal Cellular Health

Nectarine antioxidants help protect against cancer and other diseases by reducing the cellular damage that occurs when the body burns oxygen. Nectarines promote healthy red blood cell formation and fluid that regulates heart rate.

Nectarines Lower Cholesterol Levels and Promotes Digestion

The fiber in nectarines helps control blood cholesterol levels. The skins contribute to insoluble fiber which helps prevent constipation.

Nectarines Help Inhibit Asthma

Nectarine anti-inflammatory activity decreases the incidence of asthma symptoms and wheezing.

Nectarines Promote Athletic Performance

Nectarines have some of the most efficient fuel for energy production and that can be stored in muscle and liver, functioning as an energy source for prolonged, strenuous exercise. Nectarines can be used as a source to provide the most important nutrients for sports performance. Overall, emphasizing intake of fruits and other high-quality vegetables while reducing intake of fatty foods will be beneficial for athletic performance.

Anti-Cancer Benefits

Consumption of nectarines is known to lower the risk of cancer. Many doctors recommend that people wishing to reduce their risk of cancer eat several nectarines along with other servings of fruit due to their high levels of antioxidants.

Original Oranges

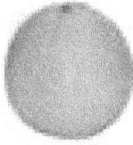

In an organic system you don't waste anything. We need to educate the consumer to accept a tiny blemish on an orange. Robert Patterson

Original Oranges

Supports the Immune system

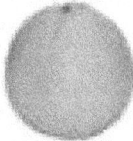

Combats cancer

Protects your heart

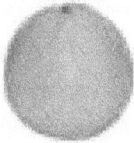

Supports Good Respiration.

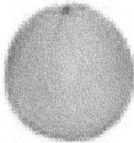

Reduces Inflammation

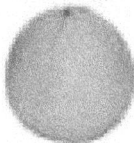

Balances Blood Sugar Levels

Health Benefits of Oranges

A diet rich in citrus consumption has been found to protect against arthritis, asthma, Alzheimer's disease and cognitive impairment, Parkinson's disease, macular degeneration, diabetes, gallstones, multiple sclerosis, cholera, gingivitis cataracts and ulcerative colitis. Oranges have phytonutrients and flavonoids which have been shown to have anti-inflammatory, anti-tumor and blood clot inhibiting properties, as well as strong antioxidant effects. Oranges are powerful in their ability to ward off sickness and disease.

Oranges have a wide variety of phytonutrients which have been shown to lower high blood pressure as well as lower cholesterol. They have also been shown to have strong anti-inflammatory properties. Importantly, most of these phytonutrients are found in the peel and inner white pulp of the orange.

Consuming oranges have been found to reduce one's risk of developing lung cancer. It has also been found that ingesting oranges daily can significantly lower your risk of developing rheumatoid arthritis. An orange a day may also help keep ulcers away.

A Healthy Dose of Oranges for Antioxidant Protection and Immune Support

You may already know that oranges are an excellent source of antioxidants in the body, disarming free radicals and preventing damage both inside and outside cells. Preventing DNA mutations translates into preventing cancer.

Oranges and a Reduction of Inflammation

Oranges prevent free radical damage that trigger an inflammatory overload associated with reduced severity of inflammatory conditions, such as asthma, osteoarthritis, and rheumatoid arthritis.

Protection against Cardiovascular Disease and Cancer

A diet that features oranges is a defense against cardiovascular disease. Oranges reduce the risk of cardiovascular factors of blood pressure, protecting against stroke and cardiac arrhythmias.

Antioxidant, Anti-viral, Anti-allergenic, Anti-inflammatory, Anti-carcinogenic

Oranges have been shown to have a wide range of antioxidant, anti-viral, anti-allergenic, anti-inflammatory, anti-proliferative and anti-carcinogenic effects.

Compounds in Orange Peel May Lower Cholesterol as Effectively as Statin Drugs

The antioxidants in citrus fruit peels have been found to have the potential to lower cholesterol more effectively than some prescription drugs, and without side effects. Grating a tablespoon or so of the peel from well-scrubbed organic oranges each day and using it to flavor tea, salads, salad dressings, yogurt, soups, hot oatmeal, buckwheat or rice may be a practical way of achieving some cholesterol-lowering benefits. The orange peel works like statin drugs, by inhibiting the synthesis of cholesterol and triglycerides inside the liver.

A Very Good Source of Fiber and Balancing Blood Sugar Levels

A single orange provides fiber, which has been shown to reduce high cholesterol levels. The fiber of oranges can help by keeping blood sugar levels under control, which explains why oranges can be a healthy snack for people with diabetes. In addition, the natural fruit sugars in oranges keep blood sugar levels from rising too high after eating. The fiber in oranges reduces the uncomfortable constipation or diarrhea in those suffering from irritable bowel syndrome.

Prevent Kidney Stones

Want to reduce your risk of calcium oxalate kidney stones? Ingest oranges. When you consume oranges your urinary pH value and citric acid excretion increases, significantly dropping your risk of forming calcium oxalate stones.

Promising Peaches

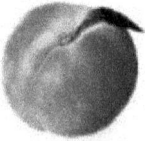

"A Georgia peach, a real Georgia peach, a backyard great-grandmother's orchard peach, is as thickly furred as a sweater, and so fluent and sweet that once you bite through the flannel, it brings tears to your eyes." ~Melissa Fay Greene, 'Praying for Sheetrock'

Promising Peaches

Prevents Constipation

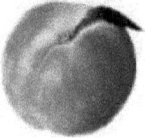

Combats Cancer

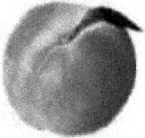

Helps stop strokes

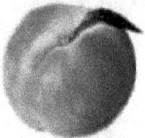

Aids Digestion

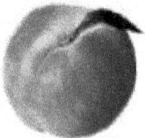

Helps hemorrhoids

Health Benefits of Peaches

Peaches are high in a number of nutrients your body needs. They are also high in antioxidants that are essential for a healthy heart and eyes. The darker the peach's color, the more antioxidants it has in its pulp.

The antioxidants may also help in maintaining healthy urinary and digestive functions. Peaches are good relief for stomach ulcers and other digestive issues like colitis and kidney disease. This is due to peaches being high in fiber.

Various ailments have been prevented or treated with some success by regular consumption of peaches, such as acidosis, anemia, asthma, bladder and kidney stones, bronchitis, constipation, dry cough, gastritis and high blood pressure.

Health benefits of peaches embrace various therapeutic properties as well as its great refreshing and nourishing actions. Peaches can be a solution to quench the thirst and recharge your body with energy.

Combat Various Digestive Problems
Peaches relieve the symptoms of gastritis, indigestion, constipation, heaviness in the stomach, flatulence and nausea. Peaches are a natural remedy to fight digestive problems caused by headaches, stresses, anxiety, menopause and other similar conditions. Consumption of peaches on a regular basis can help in regulating bowel movements and in getting rid of constipation. Peaches can be used to remove worms from the intestines.

Aids Kidney Function
Peaches are an excellent diuretic and have laxative properties; therefore, this natural product can be used to tone and stimulate the function of kidneys and bladder. Regular consumption of raw peach juice is linked to lower chances of nephritis and other diseases of the kidneys and liver. It can assist in dissolving kidney and bladder stones. Peaches also prevent fluid retention in promoting the regular flow of urine; this further alleviates gout and rheumatism to a great extent.

Support Heart Health
Peaches strengthen heart muscles and stimulate blood flow. As a result, this leads to improved blood pressure, lower cholesterol levels in blood and lower chances of atherosclerosis, myocardial infarction and other

serious cardiovascular diseases. This natural product is a great source of iron; therefore, raw peach juice benefits include protecting us against anemia.

Anti-Cancer

Peaches have powerful anti-oxidants. They help in controlling free radicals and therefore the formation of cancer cells, particularly in glands and organs with epithelial tissue. Peaches also inhibit the growth of potential tumors

Promotes Eye Health

Ingesting peaches regularly helps to prevent the formation of cataracts in your older years and helps you see better in the dark.

Protective Pears

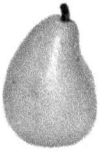

"Eating pears cleans the teeth." ~Korean proverb

Protective Pears

Promotes healthy immune system

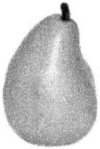

Promotes cardiovascular health

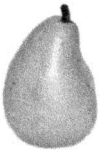

Healthy digestive system

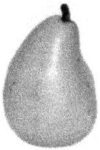

Protection against macular degeneration

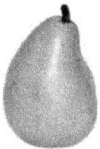

Anticancer agent

Health Benefits of Pears

Pear fiber helps prevent constipation and ensures regularity. Fiber in the colon binds to bile salts and carries them out of the body. Since bile salts are made from cholesterol, the body must break down more cholesterol to make more bile, a substance that is also necessary for digestion. The end result is a lowering of cholesterol levels. Pears promote colonic health through keeping you regular which aids in preventing colon cancer. Fiber also binds to cancer-causing chemicals in the colon, preventing them from damaging colon cells. This may be one reason why diets high in fiber-rich foods, such as pears, are associated with a reduced risk of colon cancer.

Pears Promote Healthy Eye Health
Pears may also lower your risk of age-related macular degeneration the primary cause of vision loss in older adults.

Skins of Pears are Antioxidant Rich
Antioxidant rich skins of pears help prevent cancer and artery damage that can lead to heart problems. They have also been found to protect against Alzheimer's disease. So choose to eat the peel along with your pears knowing all the benefits that you will receive!

Pears Have a Low Glycemic Index.
Pears are digested and absorbed more slowly, producing a more gradual rise in blood glucose and insulin levels. Pears help in prevention of coronary heart disease and the management of diabetes.

Cancer Prevention
The high levels of antioxidants in pears protect cells from damage by free radicals. A serving of pears a day is associated with a reduced risk of cancer in women. It has been found that eating pears help protect women against postmenopausal breast cancer.

Pears Reduce Inflammation and Promotes Healthy Breathing
Pears are useful in treating inflammation of mucous membranes, colitis, chronic gall bladder disorders, arthritis, and gout. It has been found that people who eat pears regularly have the lowest risk of developing asthma.

Digestion and Colon Health
Pears are a diuretic and have a mild laxative effect. Ingesting pears regulates bowel movement. Pears contain more fiber than many other fruits. The high fiber in pears makes them ideal for a person suffering

from constipation. Most of the fiber is insoluble, making pears a good laxative. The gritty fiber content may cut down on the number of cancerous colon polyps.

Blood Pressure
Pears have antioxidants which help prevent high blood pressure and stroke.

Sore Throat and Fever
Pears are known to have a cooling effect on the body that is excellent in relieving fever. The best way to bring a fever down quickly or sooth a sore throat is to ingest some pears. The antioxidants in pears will build your immune system so consume some pears when you feel a cold coming on.

Precious Pineapple

"The bittersweet of a white oak acorn which you nibble in a bleak November walk over the tawny earth is more to me than a slice of imported pineapple." ~Henry David Thoreau (1817-1862)

Precious Pineapple

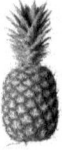

Strengthen bones

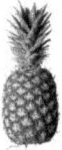

Relieves colds

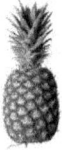

Aids congestion

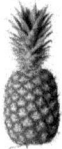

Dissolves warts

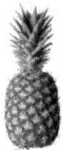

Blocks diarrhea

Pineapple Health Benefits

Pineapples are actually a composite of many flowers whose individual mini fruitlets fuse together around a central core. Each fruitlet can be identified by an "eye," which is the rough spiny marking on the pineapple's surface.

Antioxidant Protection and Immune Support

Pineapples have antioxidants that defend all areas of the body against free radicals that attack and damage normal cells. Free radicals have been shown to promote artery plaque build-up of atherosclerosis and diabetic heart disease. Pineapples have been shown to support the proper function of the immune system, making it a nutrient rich fruit to turn to for the prevention of recurrent ear infections, colds, and flu.

Strengthens Weak Bones

Pineapples are rich in phytonutrients and trace minerals that are needed for your body to build bone and connective tissues. The benefits of pineapple can effect the growth of bones in young people and the strengthening of bones in older people.

Helps Arthritis and Inflammation

Those who have arthritis pain, eating pineapples can reduce the pain of arthritis. Pineapple prevents the disease of arthritis by strengthening your bones. Bromelain is present in fresh pineapples which help in reducing the swelling in inflammatory conditions like gout, arthritis, sore throat and acute sinusitis. Also enzymes in pineapple are used for treating rheumatoid arthritis.

Promotes Healthy Tissue Repair and Circulation

Pineapples speed up the tissue repair associated with general surgery, diabetic ulcers and injuries. This fruit reduces blood clotting and aids in removing plaque from the arterial walls. People suffering from angina can consume pineapple because it enhances blood circulation in narrowed arteries.

Healthy Mouth and Throat

Pineapples are used to treat throat infections and bronchitis. The phytonutrients in pineapples are good for oral health. It also reduces periodontal disease and gingivitis.

Plentiful Plums

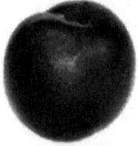

"I am putting real plums into an imaginary cake." ~ Mary McCarthy

Plentiful Plums

Plums aid in cancer prevention

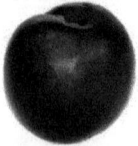

Dried plums (prunes) help restore bone mass

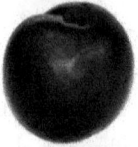

Plums and prunes are known to be an effective natural laxative

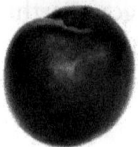

Plums help lower bad cholesterol

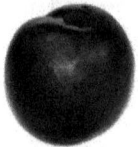

Plums aid in inhibiting cancer growth

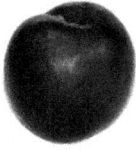

Plums have a low GI (Glycemic Index)

Plum Health Benefits

Plums contain numerous health promoting phytonutrient compounds. Plums are also high in fiber and help in supporting a healthy digestive system. Plums have high antioxidant levels which provide the body with resistance against infectious agents, counter inflammation and harmful free radicals.

Promotes Healthy Tissue Growth

Plums help maintain healthy mucus membranes and skin. Consumption of natural plums help protect from lung and oral cavity cancers.

Healthy Blood Pressure

Plums promote healthy red blood cell formation. Plums help regulate cell and body fluids that lead to stabilizing of heart rate and blood pressure.

Digestive Health

Plums are high in dietary fiber which help normalize the functions of the digestive tract and ease constipation problems.

Pungent Prunes

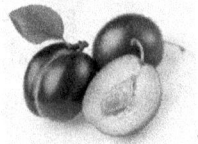

"According to the statistics, a man eats a prune every twenty seconds. I don't know who this fellow is, but I know where to find him." ~ Morey Amsterdam (1908-1966) Actor, writer, comedian

Pungent Prunes

Slows aging process

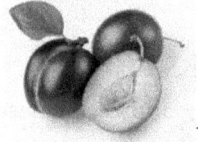

Prevents constipation

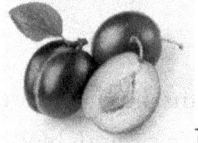

Boosts memory

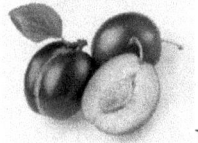

Lowers cholesterol

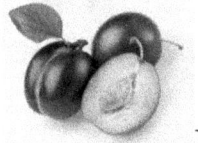

Protects against heart disease

Prune Health Benefits
Prunes help in maintaining normal blood pressure and heart function. Those diced dried prunes on top of your breakfast cereal will help to prevent high blood pressure and protect against atherosclerosis and stroke.

Promote Bone Health

Prunes counteract the increased urinary calcium loss caused by a high-salt diet, thus helping to prevent bones from thinning out at a fast rate.

Normalizing Blood Sugar Levels

Prunes' soluble fiber helps normalize blood sugar levels by slowing the rate at which food leaves the stomach and by delaying the absorption of *glucose* (the form in which sugar is transported in the blood) following a meal. Soluble fiber also increases insulin sensitivity and can therefore play a helpful role in the prevention and treatment of type 2 diabetes.

Prunes' Fiber for Regularity and Intestinal Protection

Prunes are well known for their ability to prevent constipation. In addition to providing bulk and increasing bowel movements it leads to decreasing the risk of colon cancer and hemorrhoids. Prunes' insoluble fiber provides food for the "friendly" bacteria in the large intestine. When these helpful bacteria ferment prunes' insoluble fiber, creates a reaction that serves as the primary fuel for the cells of the large intestine and helps maintain a healthy colon.

Special Strawberries

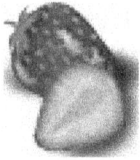

"Strawberries are the angels of the earth, innocent and sweet with green leafy wings reaching heavenward." – Terri Guillemets

Special Strawberries

Combats cancer

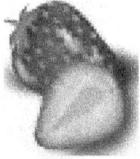

Protects your heart

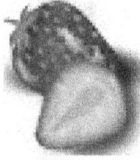

Boosts your memory

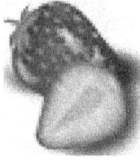

Calms Stress

Health Benefits of Strawberries

Not only do strawberries taste great they are among the fruits ranked highest in health-promoting antioxidants. Strawberry anti-inflammatory nutrients provide cardiovascular support and prevention of cardiovascular diseases and improved regulation of blood sugar. Strawberries also promote a decreased risk of type 2 diabetes, and prevention of cancer.

Improved Blood Sugar Regulation

Great news for healthy people wanting to maintain healthy blood sugar levels, and also for people with type 2 diabetes who enjoy fresh strawberries and want to enjoy them on a regular basis.

Reducing Inflammation
It has been shown that several blood markers for chronic, unwanted inflammation can be improved by regular intake of strawberries

Antioxidant and Anti-Inflammatory Phytonutrients in Strawberries
Strawberry phytonutrients actually work together in synergistic fashion to provide their cardiovascular benefits. Strawberries provide decreased oxidation of fats in the cell membranes of cells that line our blood vessels and lead to decreased levels of circulating fats in the body.

Anti-Cancer Benefits
Strawberries reduce chronic, excessive inflammation and chronic, excessive oxidative stress which are often primary factors in the development of cancer,

Anti-Aging
Strawberries have been shown to create enhanced cognitive function in the form of better object recognition. The consumption of strawberries has been found to enhance motor function in the form of better balance and coordination of movements.

Improvement of Inflammatory Bowel Problems
The anti-inflammatory substance in strawberries decrease inflammation in the digestive tract of individuals diagnosed with inflammatory bowel diseases.

Tasty Tomatoes

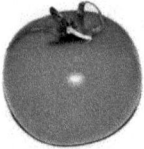

"A world without tomatoes is like a string quartet without violins."
Laurie Colwin, 'Home Cooking'

Tasty Tomatoes

Protects tomatoes

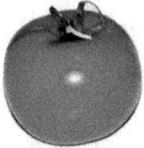

Combats cancer

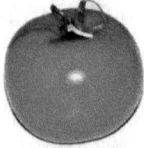

Lowers cholesterol

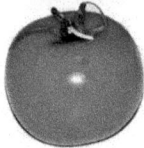

Protects your heart

Health Benefits of Tomatoes

Did you know that tomatoes are actually in the fruit family? Tomatoes are known for their outstanding antioxidant content, including, of course, their-rich concentration of lycopene. Tomatoes and their antioxidant properties have been linked to promoting bone, liver, kidneys, and bloodstream, and neurological health.

Heart Health and Cardiovascular Support

Consumption of tomatoes has been linked to heart health. Tomatoes have been shown to help lower total cholesterol, LDL cholesterol. In addition, tomato extracts have been shown to help prevent unwanted clumping together of blood cells. Tomatoes provide antioxidant support to the cardiovascular system and regulate fats in the bloodstream.

Supports Bone Health
The connection of tomato intake to bone health involves the rich supply of antioxidant in tomatoes.

Anti-Cancer Benefits
Tomatoes have repeatedly been show to provide us with anti-cancer benefits. Tomatoes are known as anti-cancer food that supplies antioxidants and anti-inflammatory nutrients to the body.

Helps to Control Diabetes:
Tomatoes have many trace minerals which help diabetics keep their blood sugar level under control.

Vision
Tomatoes are also an excellent food to help improve your vision. Tomatoes can help your eyes focus better during bouts of night blindness.

Healthy Shiny Hair:
Due to high level of antioxidants, tomatoes help keep your hair strong and shiny.

Reducing Kidney-stones and Gallstones:
Eating tomatoes without the seeds has been shown to lessen the risk of gallstones and kidney stones.

Wonderful Watermelons

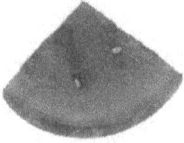

Watermelon -- it's a good fruit. You eat, you drink, and you can wash your face with it." ~Enrico Caruso

Wonderful Watermelons

Protects the prostate

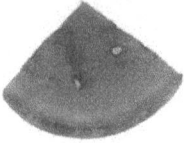

Promotes weight loss

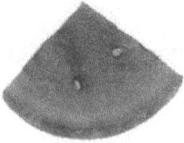

Lowers weight loss

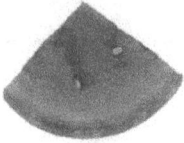

Helps stop strokes

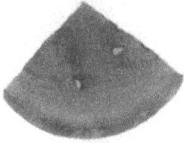

Controls blood pressure

Health Benefits of Watermelons

This delectable thirst-quencher may also help to alleviate the inflammation that contributes to conditions like asthma, atherosclerosis, diabetes, colon cancer, and arthritis. Watermelon is actually packed with some of the most important antioxidants in nature.

Anti-Cancer

Choosing to regularly eat lycopene-rich fruits, such as watermelon may greatly reduce cancer.

Watermelon Cools the Body

Watermelon is a cooling fruit that helps to remove ammonia from the body, through the cells lining our blood vessels. This causes a reaction that relaxes blood vessels, lowering high blood pressure.

Stabilizes Blood Sugar

Watermelons improve insulin sensitivity in people who have diabetes and insulin resistance.

Eat the Rainbow... A Closer Look

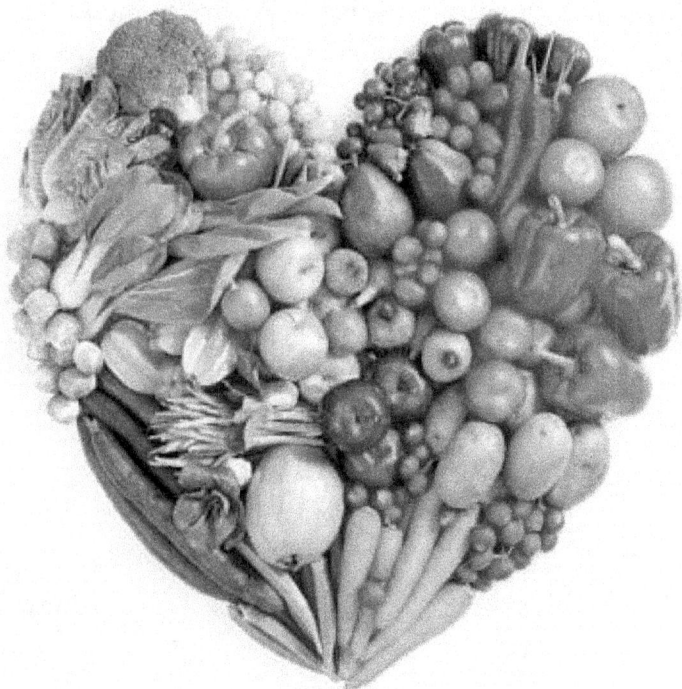

People need different amounts of fruits and vegetables depending on their age, gender and amount of daily physical activity. To learn your daily recommendation, visit www.fruitsandveggiesmatter.gov. The recommended daily amount of fruits and vegetables according to the USDA is half your plate should be filled with fruits and vegetables each and every meal.

Eat the Rainbow!

Different colored fruits & vegetables are full of nutrients. Eating a variety of these helps your body stay healthy.

Adapted from Healthy Hawaii Initiative's Eat a Rainbow Handout

GREEN

Helps your body...
- Lower your chance of getting cancer
- Keep your eyes healthy
- Keep your bones & teeth strong

You should try:
spinach, bok choy, honeydew, green peas, cucumbers, green grapes, green beans, endamame, green apples, broccoli, cauliflower, limes, cabbage, watercress, avocados

YELLOW & ORANGE

Helps your body...
- Keep your heart healthy
- Keep your eyes healthy
- Lower your chance of getting cancer
- Keep you from catching colds

You should try:
carrots, pineapple, mangoes, sweet potatoes, corn, oranges, yellow peppers, cantaloupes, lemons, pumpkins, tangerines

RED

Helps your body...
- Keep your heart healthy
- Keep your bladder healthy
- Keep your memory strong
- Lower your chance of getting cancer

You should try:
tomatoes, strawberries, red onion, red peppers, cherries, red apples, red cabbage, watermelon

BLUE & PURPLE

Helps your body...
- Stay healthy when you get old
- Keep your memory strong
- Keep your bladder healthy
- Lower your chance of getting cancer

You should try:
eggplant, blueberries, purple cabbage, purple grapes, raisins, Okinawan sweet potato (purple potato)

WHITE

Helps your body...
- Keep your heart healthy
- Have good cholesterol levels
- Lower your chance of getting cancer

You should try:
onion, chives, mushrooms, green onion, ginger, jicama

Eat the Rainbow is a chart that depicts brief examples of different fruits and vegetables from each color based on natural plant pigments. Bases for their antioxidant and phytonutrient super food abilities are also discussed.

Red Fruits and Vegetables

*Red apples *Beets *Red cabbage *Cherries *Cranberries *Pink *Grapefruit *Red grapes *Red peppers *Pomegranates *Red potatoes *Radishes *Raspberries *Rhubarb *Strawberries *Tomatoes *Watermelon

Red fruits and vegetables are colored by natural plant pigments called "lycopene" and "anthocyanins." Eating fruits and vegetables that are lycopene rich have been shown to reduce the incidence of cancer.

Eating fruits and vegetables that have the antioxidant anthocyanin act as powerful antioxidants that protect cells from damage.

Orange and Yellow Fruits and Vegetables

*Yellow apples *Apricots *Butternut squash *Cantaloupe *Carrots *Grapefruit *Lemons *Mangoes *Nectarines *Oranges *Papayas *Peaches *Pears *Yellow peppers *Persimmons *Pineapple *Pumpkin *Rutabagas *Yellow summer or winter squash *Sweet corn *Sweet potatoes *Tangerines *Yellow tomatoes *Yellow watermelon

Orange and yellow fruits and vegetables are colored by natural plant pigments called "carotenoids. Eating carotenoid-rich foods can help reduce risk of cancer, heart disease and can improve immune system function.

People who eat carotenoid-rich vegetables were found to develop less age-related macular degeneration, an eye disorder common among the elderly, which can lead to blindness. Carotenoids are good for your heart.

Citrus fruits have high amounts of folate, which will help reduce risk of birth defects.

Green Fruits and Vegetables

*Green apples *Artichokes *Asparagus *Avocados *Green beans *Broccoli *Brussels sprouts *Green cabbage *Cucumbers *Green grapes *Honeydew melon *Kiwi *Lettuce *Limes *Green onions *Peas *Green pepper *Spinach *Zucchini

Green fruits and vegetables are colored by natural plant pigment called chlorophyll and antioxidants called lutein and indoles.

Lutein keeps eyes healthy. Together, these chemicals help reduce risk of cataracts and age-related macular degeneration, which leads to blindness if untreated.

Indoles in green fruits and cruciferous vegetables help protect against some types of cancer.

Blue/Purple Fruits and Vegetables

*Blackberries *Blueberries *Eggplant *Figs *Plums *Prunes *Purple grapes *Raisins

Blue/purple fruits and vegetables are colored by natural plant pigments called anthocyanins.

Anthocyanins are antioxidants that protect cells from damage and help reduce risk of cancer, stroke and heart disease.

Eating blue and purple fruits have been shown to improve memory in regards to healthy aging.

White Fruits and Vegetables

*Bananas *Cauliflower *Garlic *Ginger *Mushrooms *Onions
*Parsnips *Potatoes *Turnips

White fruits and vegetables are colored by pigments called anthoxanthins and allicin.

Allicin helps lower cholesterol, blood pressure, reduces risk of stomach cancer and heart disease.

Eat as many of the fruits and vegetables from each color group daily. Your body will LOVE you for it!

Vegetables that Heal the Body

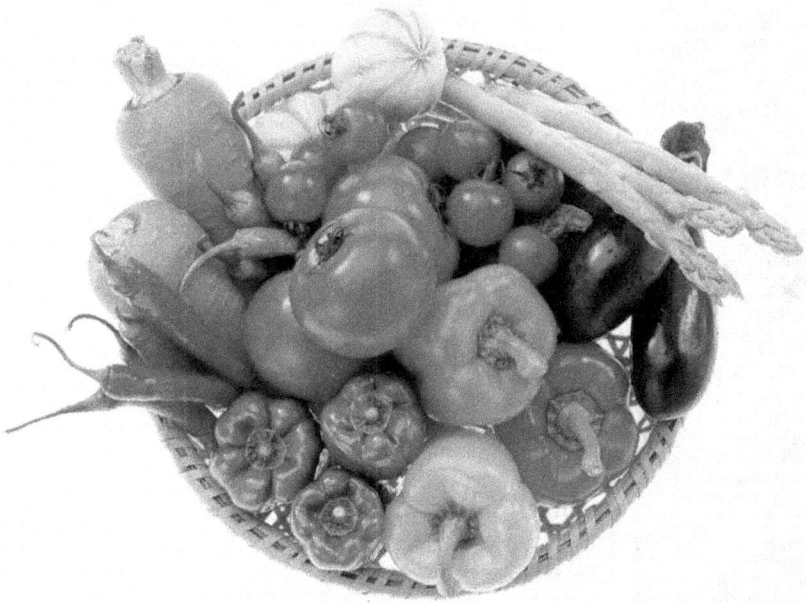

Artsy Artichokes

"His memoir is a splendid artichoke of anecdotes, in which not merely the heart and leaves but the thistles as well are edible." - John Leonard

Artsy Artichokes

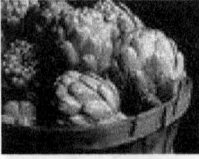 Aids digestion

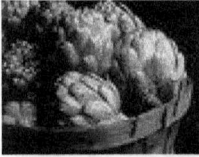 Lowers cholesterol

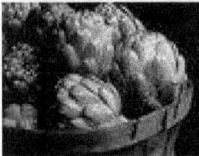 Protects your heart

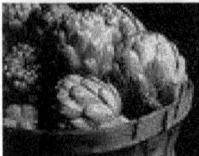 Stabilizes blood sugar

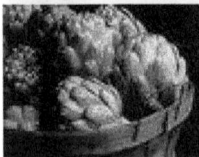 Guards against liver disease

Artichoke Health Benefits

Artichokes have trace minerals that have been found to be helpful in controlling high blood pressure. Artichokes are actually the immature flower of the thistle plant which provides protection against skin cancer. Pregnant women especially benefit from eating artichokes due to their extraordinary amounts of folate which is known for its importance in fetal development.

Promotes Healthy Liver and Digestion

Artichokes promote liver health and soothe digestive issues such as nausea, pain, and bloating. The antioxidants boost liver function by stimulating cell regeneration and scavenging for free radicals. In addition, it helps the liver cope with toxicity. Artichokes promote the liver's bile production, which in turn helps break down fatty foods.

High in Fiber

Artichokes are high in dietary fiber. The dietary fiber in artichokes help control constipation conditions, decrease bad or "LDL" cholesterol levels by binding it in the intestines and help prevent colon cancer risks by preventing toxic compounds in the food from absorption.

Helps to synthesize DNA

Artichoke enzymes help in the synthesis of DNA and optimum cellular metabolic functions.

Anti-aging

Artichokes are one of the vegetable sources which provide for bone health by promoting bone formation activity. Artichokes also help in limiting neural damage in the brain and has established a role in the treatment of patients suffering from Alzheimer's disease.

Healthy Heart and Blood Pressure

Artichokes have components that regulate body fluids and help control heart rate and blood pressure.

Attractive Asparagus

"You needn't tell me that a man who doesn't love asparagus and good wine has got a soul or a stomach either. He's simply got the instinct for being unhappy."
~'Saki', pen name of Scottish writer Hector Hugh Munro (1870-1916)

Attractive Asparagus

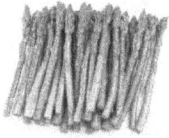

Anti-inflammatory

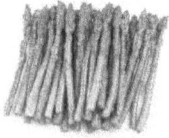

Improved blood pressure

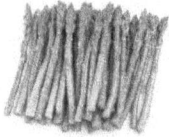

Digestive support

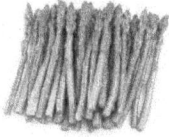

Heart health

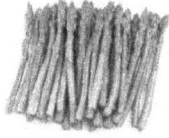

Blood sugar regulation

Health Benefits of Asparagus

Asparagus has been shown to have anti-inflammatory and anti-cancer properties and their intake has also been associated with improved blood pressure, improved blood sugar regulation, and better control of blood fat levels. Asparagus antioxidants promote digestive qualities such as nutrient absorption, lower risk of allergy, and lower the risk of colon cancer.

Digestive Support

Asparagus has high fiber content and contains a noteworthy amount of protein. Both fiber and protein help stabilize our digestion and keep food moving through us at the desirable rate.

Detoxifies the System

Asparagus has a substantial amount of fiber which cleanses the digestive system.

Anti-aging

Asparagus has antioxidants that protect cells from toxins and free radicals.

Preventing osteoporosis and osteoarthritis

Asparagus antioxidants have been shown to prevent osteoporosis. These antioxidants also aid in bone formation and tissue repair.

Promotes Healthy Urinary Tract

The consumption of asparagus helps prevent and treat urinary tract infection and kidney stones.

Awesome Avocados

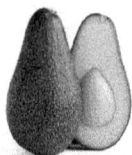

The avocado is a food without rival among the fruits, the veritable fruit of paradise.
~ David Fairchild

Awesome Avocados

Battles diabetes

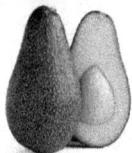

Lowers cholesterol

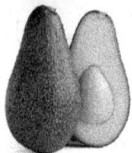

Helps stop strokes.

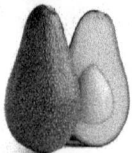

Controls blood pressure

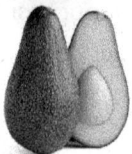

Smoothes skin

Avocado Health Benefits

The method you use to peel an avocado can make a difference to your health. Research has shown that the greatest concentration of antioxidants in avocado is in the dark green flesh that lies just beneath the skin. You do not want to slice into that dark green portion any more than necessary when you are peeling an avocado. The best method is actually end up peeling the avocado with your hands in the same way that you would peel a banana.

Fat of Avocados Act as an Anti-Inflammatory in the Body
While it is true that avocado is a high-fat food, the fat contained in avocado is unusual and provides research-based health benefits. Avocados have phytonutrients that are supporters of our system that help keep inflammation under control. The anti-inflammatory benefits of these avocado fats are particularly well-documented with problems involving arthritis. Over half of the total fat in avocado is provided in the form of oleic acid—very similar to the fat composition of olives and olive oil.

Fat of Avocados Promote a Healthy Digestive System
Oleic acid helps our digestive tract form transport molecules for fat that can increase our absorption of fat-soluble nutrients. As a monounsaturated fatty acid, it has also been shown to help lower our risk of heart disease.

Anti-Cancer Defense
Antioxidants and phytonutrients in avocados have been found to seek out pre-cancerous and cancer cells then destroy them without harming healthy cells.

Eye Health
Avocados protect against macular degeneration and cataract of the eyes.

Lower Cholesterol
Avocados have compounds that have been shown to lower cholesterol levels.

Heart Health
Avocados help regulate blood flow and have been shown to promote heart health and stroke prevention.

Better Nutrient Absorption
It has been found that certain nutrients are absorbed better when eaten with avocado.

Bountiful Beans

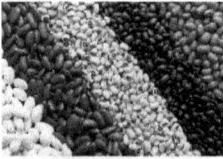

"Beans are highly nutritious and satisfying, they can also be delicious if and when properly prepared. They possess over all vegetables the great advantage of being just as good, if not better, when kept waiting, an advantage in the case of people whose disposition or occupation makes it difficult for them to be punctual at mealtime." Andre Simon (1877-1970) The Concise Encyclopedia of Gastronomy' (1952)

Bountiful Beans

Promotes healthy digestion

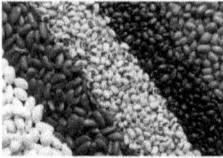

Prevents bowel movement problems

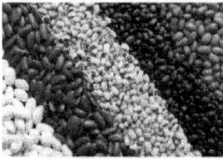

Helps hemorrhoids

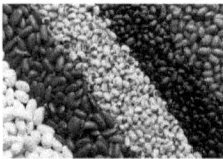

Lowers cholesterol

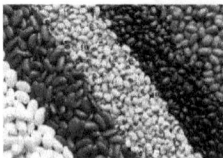

Combats cancer

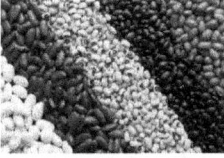

Improve diabetics' blood glucose control

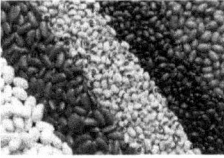

Reduce risk of many cancers

Health Benefits of Beans

Beans belong to an extremely large category of vegetables, containing more than 13,000 species which are known to provide the health benefits of plant based proteins to the world's population. Beans offer a high rate of antioxidant protection. The health benefits of beans are astounding. The antioxidants and the phytonutrients of beans have been know to ease the symptoms of menopause, prevent cancer, reduce risk of heart disease and improve bone health.

Beans are a Rich Source of Fiber

When you eat beans, they are not entirely digested, so the undigested material resides in the colon, where bacteria attack it and start to feed on it.

In the process, lots of chemicals are released, which tell your liver to cut down its production of cholesterol and your blood to speed up clearing out dangerous LDL cholesterol. Plus, fiber can actually mop up cholesterol from the intestine and clear it out of the system.

Chemicals that block formation of cancer cells are released. In fact, beans are concentrated carriers of enzymes that counteract the activation of cancer-causing compounds in the colon.

Controls PMS

Beans have been shown to produce fewer cramps and mood swings in women who are prone to PMS.

Protect your Heart

The soluble fiber found in beans help to reduce LDL or bad cholesterol levels. Plus, it has been shown to reduce inflammation and blood pressure which is beneficial for heart health.

Beans Boost Your Enzymes

Beans boost enzymes in making skin pigment and connective tissues.

Better Beets

"Everything I do, I do on the principle of Russian borscht. You can throw everything into it beets, carrots, cabbage, onions, everything you want. What's important is the result, the taste of the borscht." ~Yevgeny Yevtushenko, Russian poet

Better Beets

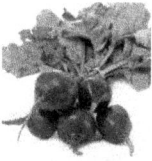

Controls blood pressure

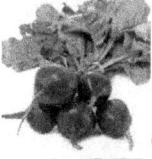

Combats cancer

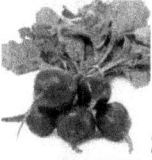

Strengthens bones

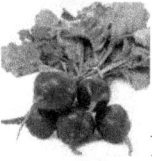

Protects your heart

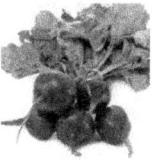

Aids weight loss

Health Benefits of Beets

Beets are a unique source of phytonutrients and have been shown to provide antioxidant, anti-inflammatory, and detoxification support. When red beets are eaten regularly they help against certain oxidative stress-related disorders.

Anti-Cancer and Red Beets:

Beet root is a traditional treatment used for leukemia. Beet root contains antioxidants and phytonutrients which have anti-cancer properties.

Sharper Eyes

Beets support eye health and common age-related eye problems involving the macula and the retina.

Reduce Cholesterol

Fiber in red beets help reduce serum cholesterol.

Promotes Healthy Blood Pressure and Circulatory System

Beets can help in normalizing blood pressure. When consumed regularly beets help promote the elasticity of arteries to prevent varicose veins. Beets are also a powerful cleanser and builder of blood.

Detoxification and Cleansing

Beets help stimulate the function of liver cells and protect the liver and bile ducts. Beets are highly alkaline which makes it effective for those who have acidosis.

Healthy Digestive System

Regular beet consumption relieves constipation. Beets when ingested regularly assist in healing gout, kidney and gall bladder problems.

Bountiful Broccoli

"Fatherhood is telling your daughter that movie stars love all their fans, but they especially have special feelings for the ones who eat broccoli." Bill Cosby, 'Fatherhood' (1986)

Bountiful Broccoli

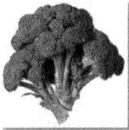
Strengthens bones

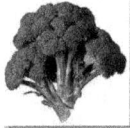
Saves eyesight

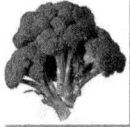
Combats cancer

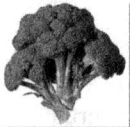
Protects your heart

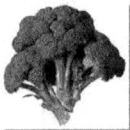
Controls blood pressure

Health Benefits of Broccoli

When broccoli is steamed it can provide you with some special cholesterol-lowering benefits if you will cook it by steaming. The fiber-related components in broccoli do a better job of binding together with bile acids in your digestive tract when they have been steamed. Broccoli positively impacts the body's detoxification system which supports all steps in body's detox process, including activation, neutralization, and elimination of unwanted contaminants.

Healthy Eyes
Broccoli contains phytonutrient antioxidants that promote the health of the lenses of the eyes.

Strong Bones
Studies have shown that **(broccoli contains more calcium than most dairy products)** therefore helping to build bone mass.

Relieves Colds
The antioxidant and anti-inflammatory benefits help relieve cold symptoms.

Healthy Nervous system
Broccoli contains high amounts of phytonutrients that help in optimal functioning of brain, to maintain healthy nervous system and promotes regular growth of muscles.

Blood Pressure
The phytonutrients and antioxidants in broccoli regulate blood pressure.

Skin Health
Broccoli helps in repairing skin damage that detoxifies and repairs the skin itself.

Strong Heart
Prevents thickening of arteries in human body, which leads to preventing heart disease and stroke.

Diabetes
Due to its high fiber content and low sugar, broccoli helps keep blood sugar low and as a result insulin can be kept to a minimum.

Caring Cabbage

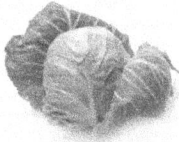

"The old Romans having expelled physicians out of their commonwealth did for many years maintain their health by the use of cabbages, eating them for every disease." ~16th Century Historian

Caring Cabbage

Combats cancer

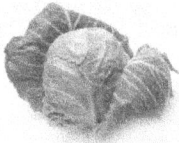

Prevents constipation

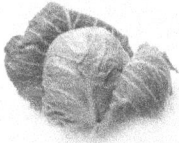

Promotes weight loss

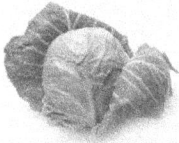

Protects your heart

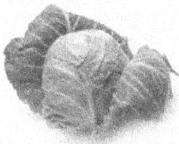

Helps hemorrhoids

Cabbage has many known healing properties. Cabbage is considered to be highly healthy. In fact, the health benefits of cabbage dates back to ancient times where Greeks used cabbage to heal eye infections.

Anti-Cancer
Cabbage fights cancer risks

Aids Healthy Digestion

Cabbage is fiber-laden which aids digestion, water absorption and eases defecation.

Heart Health

The antioxidants and phytonutrients in cabbage ensure nerve and heart health.

Youthful Clear Skin

Cabbage provides phytonutrients that provide youthful and clear skin. The antioxidants in cabbage protect the skin against aging fast.

Boosts the Production of Antibodies

Cabbage boosts the immune system and aids in building antibodies in the body.

Cute Carrots

"Some like carrots, others like cabbage. Some like carrots with cabbage." ~ Anonymous

Cute Carrots

Health Benefits of Carrots

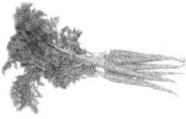

Saves eyesight

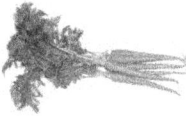

Protects your heart

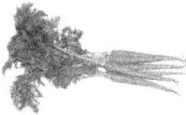

Prevents constipation

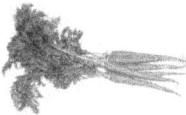

Combats cancer

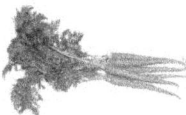

Promotes weight loss

Health Benefits of Carrots

Your mother may have told you that carrots will make your eyes sharper, but that is not the only power of carrots. Carrots have many antioxidant and phytonutrient compounds. Some antioxidants in carrots have been found to help the immune system to target and destroy cancer cells in the body. It also prevents DNA variation and fat oxidation that ultimately protect cells against free radicals.

Carrots assist in preventing the narrowing of blood vessels resulting from contracting of the muscular wall of the vessels. This in turn promotes regular heartbeat and healthy metabolism.

Promotes Healthy Digestion
Regular consumption of carrots provides for healthy functioning of the liver and digestive tract.

Ache Relief Due to Aging
Carrots help in the relief process of aches due to aging and helps strengthen bones.

Promotes Good Cholesterol
Helps lower bad LDL cholesterol throughout the body.

Detoxification and Cleansing
Regular consumption of carrots reduces fat and bile in the liver.

Healthy Glowing Skin
The antioxidants and orange natural pigment of carrots provides for the skins healthy glow and prevents cell degeneration.

Colorful Cauliflower

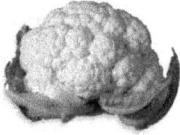

"Cauliflower is nothing but a cabbage with a college education."~ Mark Twain

Colorful Cauliflower

Protects against prostate cancer

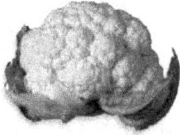

Combats breast cancer

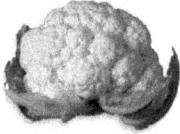

Strengthens bones

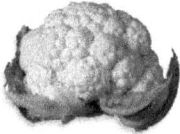

Banishes bruises

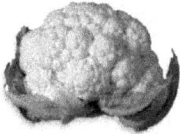

Guards against heart disease

Health Benefits of Cauliflower

Cauliflower is an excellent source of antioxidants and phytonutrients. It is also a good source of fiber. Cauliflower is a part of the cruciferous family of vegetables that help prevent cancer. The cancer fighting agents help to increase the activity of enzymes that disable and eliminate carcinogens.

Anti-Inflammation

Cauliflower contains phytonutrients and omega-3 fatty acids that decrease inflammation. Potentially, regular cauliflower consumption can help decrease the risk of inflammation-mediated diseases.

Healthy Cardiovascular System

By virtue of having antioxidant and anti-inflammatory properties, cauliflower consumption is protective against cardiovascular and cerebrovascular diseases.

Digestive System and Detoxification

Cauliflower is high in dietary fiber, which helps clean your digestive system and gets rid of unnecessary substances. Cauliflower also promotes positive growth of your stomach lining which wards off unhealthy bacteria.

Courageous Celery

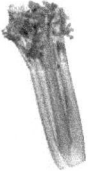

"Good cooking does not depend on whether the dish is large or small, expensive or economical. If one has the art, then a piece of celery or salted cabbage can be made into a marvelous delicacy; whereas if one has not the art, not all the greatest delicacies and rarities of land, sea or sky are of any avail." ~Yuan Mei

Courageous Celery

Promotes healthy immune system

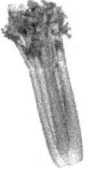

Lowers blood pressure

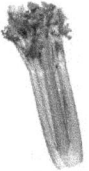

Provides healthy bowel movement

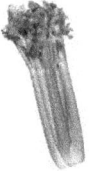

Provides healthy sodium

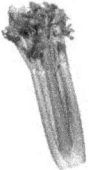

Combats cancer

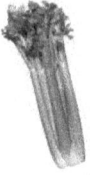

Normalize blood pressure

Health Benefits of Celery
Nutrients and fiber in celery aid in producing a healthy digestive system. The natural organic sodium (salt) in celery is more easily digested through consumption and is essential for the body. Even individuals who are salt-sensitive can safely take the sodium in celery, unlike table salt (iodized sodium) which is harmful for those with high blood pressure.

Healthy Blood Pressure
Celery has always been associated with lowering of blood pressure due to its natural sodium content and how it is processed by the body. Celery also helps relax the muscle around arteries, dilating the vessels and allows blood to flow normally.

Lowers Acidity:
Antioxidants and phytonutrients in celery effectively balance the body's blood pH, neutralizing acidity.

Pre/Post Workout Snack
Celery is a great pre/post work out snack because it replaces lost electrolytes and rehydrates the body with its rich minerals.

Anti-Cancer
Celery is known to contain anti-cancer compounds which help to stop the growth of tumor cells. The antioxidants and phytonutrients help prevent free radicals from damaging cells.

Lowers Cholesterol
Celery has been shown to effectively lower total cholesterol and LDL (bad) cholesterol.

Relieves Constipation

Celery can be used as a natural laxative to relieve constipation. It also helps relax nerves that have been overworked by man-made laxatives.

Cooling the Body

During dry and hot weather ingesting celery will help to normalize body temperature.

Natural Diuretic

The natural sodium in celery helps to regulate body fluid and stimulate urine production, making it important to rid the body of excess fluid.

Inflammation

The antioxidants and phytonutrients in celery help the relief of inflammation in the body.

Kidney function

Celery promotes healthy and normal kidney function by aiding elimination of toxins from the body. While eliminating toxins, it also prevents formation of kidney stones.

Calms Nervous system

The antioxidants and phytonutrients in celery juice have a calming effect on the nervous system, making it a wonderful calming juice for insomniacs.

Confident Collards

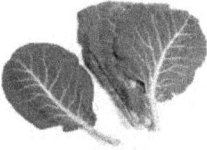

Collard greens are like flowers added to a lovely bouquet when I add them to my recipe. ~ Southern cook.

Confident Collards

Controls cholesterol

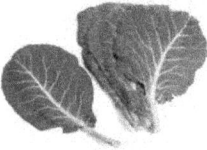

Provides healthy bowel movement

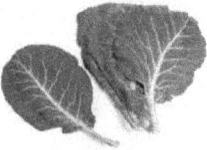

Anticancer

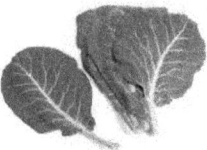

Provides healthy immune system

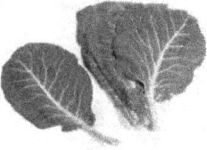

Antiviral and antibacterial

Health Benefits of Collard Greens

Collard Greens are considered good for health because of their high antioxidant and phytonutrient compounds. These phytonutrients or phytochemicals are important for providing protection against many deadly diseases. Health benefits of collard greens are primarily associated with three important benefits: antioxidant, anti-inflammatory and promotion of the body detox system.

Digestion and Detoxification Support

The phytonutrients in collard greens help to get rid of toxins from the body. The dietary fibers in this cruciferous vegetable protect the stomach lining from over growth of bad bacteria.

Cancer prevention

The phytonutrients and the anti-inflammatory compounds in collard greens help in supporting the detoxification and anti-inflammatory systems of the body thus reducing cancer risk. Collard Greens also combat cancer through reducing oxidative stress.

Healthy Cardiovascular System

Dark green leafy vegetables are always great food for the heart. It is said that collard greens are the best cruciferous vegetable for lowering cholesterol levels. They bind the bile acid and help the excretion of it. Bile acids are made from cholesterol and by flushing them out from the body; which actually lowers the cholesterol levels in the body.

Bone Health

Consumption of collard greens will help promote bone mass and make bones stronger.

Creative Corn

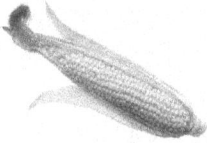

A light wind swept over the corn, and all nature laughed in the sunshine. ~A Day in the Country

Creative Corn

High in antioxidants

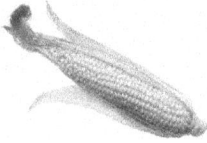

Promotes good digestion

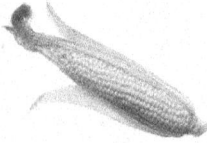

Blood sugar benefits

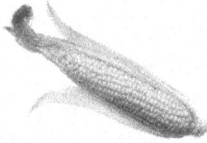

High in fiber

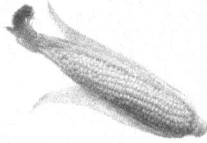

Promotes good heart health

* For the purposes of this book the corn health benefits being described are in reference to NON Genetically Modified corn.

Health Benefits of Corn

Health benefits of corn include controlling diabetes and prevention of heart ailments. Corn has been known to lower hypertension. Corn is high in fiber which aids in healthy digestion. Corn is rich in antioxidants and phytochemicals that aid in protection against chronic disease. Corn also promotes nerve health and cognitive function.

Lowers Bad Cholesterol

Consumption of corn has been found to lower plasma LDL cholesterol by reducing cholesterol absorption in the body. Corn has the effect of lowering cholesterol levels thus reducing the risk of cardiovascular disease. Even the fiber content lowers the cholesterol levels.

Protects against Diabetes and Hypertension

The phytochemicals in corn protect against diabetes and hypertension. Corn's fiber content reduces blood sugar levels for diabetic patients.

Healthy Skin

Cosmetic benefits are one of the benefits of corn. Corn starch is used in various cosmetics and is also applied topically to provide the soothing effect on skin rashes and irritation.

Healthy Digestive System

The fiber content of one cup of corn aids in alleviating digestive problems such as constipation and hemorrhoids, as well as lowering the risk of colon cancer.

Antioxidant Properties of Corn

Corn is a rich source of antioxidants which fight cancer causing free radicals. In fact, cooking increases the antioxidants in sweet corn.

Cool Cucumbers

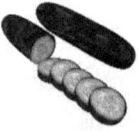

As for myself, I am sitting up today for the first time - partly dressed as the cucumber said when oil & vinegar were poured over him salt & pepper being omitted." Edward Lear, English artist, writer; 'literary nonsense' (1812-1888)

Cool Cucumbers

Reduced risk of cancer

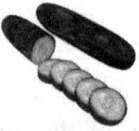

Promotes heart health

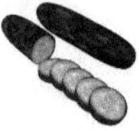

Anti-inflammatory

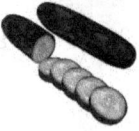

Helps keep the body hydrated.

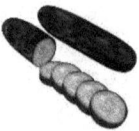

Helps regulate the body's inner core temperature,

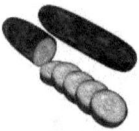

Helps flush the body of toxins.

Health Benefits of Cucumbers

Cucumbers are 95% water; they keep the body hydrated and help regulate the body's inner temperature. They also help the body flush out toxins. When you ingest cucumbers with the skin after it has been thoroughly washed you will receive higher amounts of the phytonutrients and antioxidants that it possesses.

Cosmetic Appeal

The skin of cucumbers can be used to relieve sunburn and mild skin irritations, similar to aloe vera. When cucumbers are placed on the eyes they are known to relieve puffiness.

Digestion and Detoxification

Cucumber is a natural diuretic known to promote the flow of urine. Cucumbers help in promoting a healthy liver, kidneys and pancreas.

Regulate Blood Pressure

Cucumbers are useful for regulating high and low blood pressure.

Healthy Nails

The high mineral content of cucumbers helps to prevent splitting nails of fingers and toes.

Elegant Eggplant

How can people say they don't eat eggplant when God loves the color and the French love the name? I don't understand."~ Jeff Smith (The Gourmet)

Elegant Eggplant

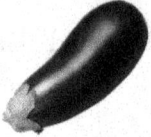

Promotes cardiovascular health

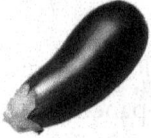

Brain food

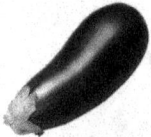

Stabilizes blood sugar

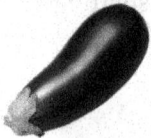

High in fiber

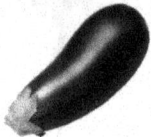

Anticancer

Health Benefits of Eggplant

Eggplant has a high source of dietary fiber and potassium. Eggplant is a potent antioxidant and free-radical scavenger. Eggplant has a low glycemic index and has been used as a source for diabetes and hypertension management.

Healthy Heart

Eggplants can help lower blood cholesterol levels and also blood pressure, thus lessening the risk of heart disease. Eggplants help keep the body hydrated to the correct levels, thus avoiding fluid retention, which can contribute to coronary heart disease.

Healthy Brain

Eggplant protects the cell membranes in the brain from damage and assists the transmission of messages from the brain to other parts of the body. Thus egg plants aids memory and brain function.

Healthy Digestion

Eggplant's high fiber content helps to keep the digestive system working well, and ease constipation.

Glorious Garlic

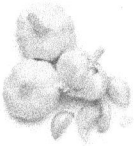

Garlic used as it should be used is the soul, the divine essence, of cookery. The cook who can employ it successfully will be found to possess the delicacy of perception, the accuracy of judgment, and the dexterity of hand which go to the formation of a great artist."~Mrs. W. G. Waters in 'The Cook's Decameron,' 1920

Glorious Garlic

Lowers cholesterol

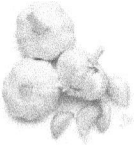

Controls blood pressure

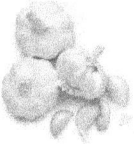

Combats cancer

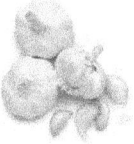

Kills bacteria

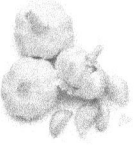

Fights fungus

Health Benefits of Garlic

Garlic has anti-viral, anti-bacterial, anti-oxidant and anti-fungal properties. Garlic can be used to build immunity due to its anti-bacterial, anti-viral properties.

Regulate Blood Sugar

Garlic can be helpful for diabetes patients because it can increase the release of insulin in blood and thus regulate blood sugar levels.

Regulate Blood Pressure

Ingesting garlic on a daily basis helps to lower high blood pressure.

Cancer Prevention

The antioxidants and phytonutrients in garlic are found to be neutralizers for compounds that cause cancer.

Healthy Digestion

Garlic helps to stimulate the secretion of digestive juices in the stomach and helps with elimination of waste material in the stomach.

Healthy Heart

Garlic has been known to help control blood pressure which leads to a healthy heart and the prevention of strokes.

Kicking Kale

"There are two types of people; those who eat kale and those who should." ~ Bo
Muller-Moore

Kicking Kale

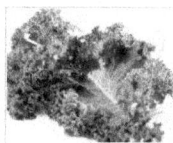 High in antioxidants.

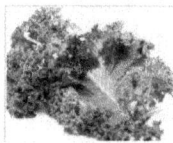 Anti-inflammatory

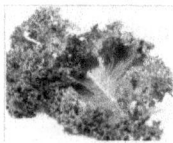 Anticancer

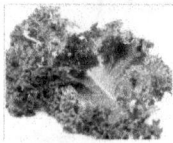 Provides cardiovascular support

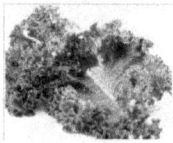 Helps detoxify the body

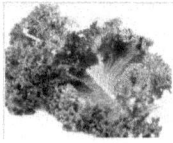 Boosts immunity

Health Benefits of Kale

Kale contains high amounts of phytochemicals and antioxidants that
act as anti-cancer properties that prevent the growth of carcinogenic
cells. Kale helps in strengthening your bones and promotes general
bone health.

Eye Health

Kale has light-filtering functions that protect the eye. This in turn prevents retinal detachment and also protects against age-related loss of vision that leads to macular degeneration.

Healthy Heart

The high amount of fiber that is present in kale helps in lowering the cholesterol level in the body which reduces the chances of having heart diseases. Kale also helps lower blood pressure that leads to a healthy cardio-vascular system.

Boosts Body Resistance

Kale is a natural antioxidant that aids the body in developing resistance against infections and gets rid of harmful oxygen free radicals.

Healthy Brain

It helps in controlling the neuronal damage to the brain,

Luscious Leeks

"Eat leeks in March and wild garlic in May and all year after physicians may play." ~Old Welsh Rhyme

Luscious Leeks

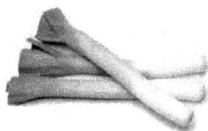

Cardiovascular support

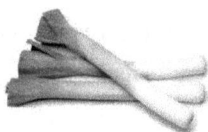

Supports blood sugar stability

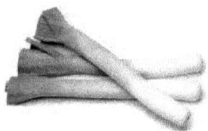

Anticancer

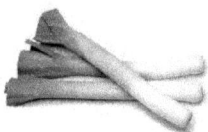

Laxative quality

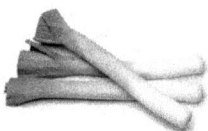

Anti-arthritic properties

Health Benefits of Leeks

Leek can help fight various types of anemia, especially those resulting from iron deficiency. Due to its anti-inflammatory and anti-septic properties, leek can be used to ward off inflammation in the body.

Healthy Digestion

Leeks are high in fiber and can be used to help regulate intestinal function. Leeks also help to repopulate the good bacteria in the colon, thereby aiding digestion and reducing intestinal bloating.

Regulate Blood Pressure and Reduces High Cholesterol

Leeks help to regulate blood pressure. Leek has anti-cholesterol and anti-atherosclerosis action. It helps reduce both the absorption of cholesterol from the intestine, as well as the oxidation of LDL-cholesterol in the blood.

Healthy Nervous System

Leeks help improve concentration, memory and the brain's ability to process information.

Detoxification

Perhaps the most characteristic action of leek juice is its purifying effect on the whole body, since it helps eliminate toxins from the body by enhancing the cleansing of the colon.

Regal Romaine Lettuce

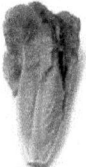

"Lettuce! O Lettuce! Let us, O let us, O Lettuce leaves, O let us leave this tree and eat Lettuce, and O let us. Lettuce leaves!" Edward Lear, English artist, writer (1812-1888) 'The History of the Seven Families of the Lake Pipple-Popple'

Regal Romaine Lettuce

Cardiovascular support

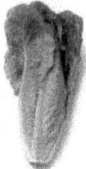

Lowers cholesterol

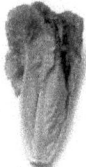

Stabilizes blood pressure

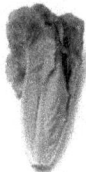

Anticancer

Health Benefits of Romaine Lettuce

Romaine lettuce contains antioxidants and phytonutrients that act as a tranquilizer and pain reducer associated with the problems of sleeplessness, anxiety and nervous disorders. Not all lettuce is created equal, but if you start your meal with a salad made of romaine lettuce you will be sure to add not only a variety of textures and flavors to your meal but an enormous amount of nutritional value. In general, the darker the leaf is the greater the nutrient content and a good source of chlorophyll.

Healthy Heart

Romaine lettuce helps prevent oxidation of cholesterol. Romaine helps to prevent plaque from building on the artery walls due to oxidation of cholesterol.

Fights Anemia

Romaine is high in chlorophyll. The chlorophyll in romaine lettuce binds easily with iron and is essential for the synthesis of hemoglobin in red blood cells.

High in Anti-oxidants

The antioxidants in romaine lettuce keeps the body clean of toxins. Romaine lettuce also aids in preventing damage caused by free radicals that create premature aging. Romaine lettuce also reduces the risk of other chronic diseases and cancer.

Outstanding Onions

"The onion and its satin wrappings are among the most beautiful of vegetables and is the only one that represents the essence of things. It can be said to have a soul."
~ Charles Dudley Warner, 'My Summer in a Garden' (1871)

Outstanding Onions

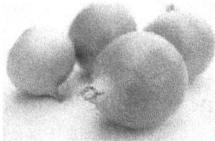

Reduce risk of heart attack

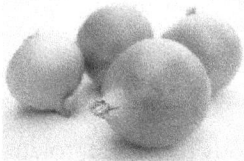

Combats cancer

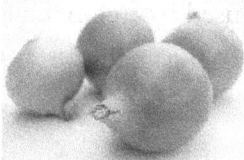

Kills bacteria

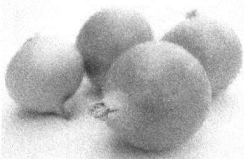

Lowers cholesterol

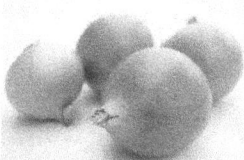

Fights fungus

Health Benefits of Onions

Onions are a powerful anti-septic. Onions have a high content of iron that makes it beneficial for warding off anemia. Onions act as an anti-inflammatory agent in the body.

Onions act as antiseptic agents that can fight different infection and bacteria including E.coli and salmonella.

Immune Booster
Onion is useful in cold weather to defend against infections, reduce fever and sweat out colds and flu.

Regulate Blood Pressure
Onions can help you to reduce blood pressure naturally whether you are eating it raw or cooked. It will dissolve blood clots and clear unhealthy fats of blood.

Anti-Coagulant
If you are eating half of a medium raw onion daily, it significantly helps to lower LDL cholesterol and prevents heart attacks.

Cancer Prevention:
Onion can arouse the growth of good bacteria in the colon. The phytonutrients and antioxidants help to reduce the risk of tumors developing in the colon.

Constipation and Flatulence
The use of plenty of onion in cooking helps to relieve chronic constipation and flatulence.

Regulate Blood Sugar
Onion helps diabetic cells to respond in bringing down the insulin level and improve glucose tolerance.

Diuretic and Blood Cleansing
Onions can help in countering fluid retention.

Urinary Tract Health
Anti-bacterial properties of onions help to remove bacteria that cause infection.

Gracious Green Peas

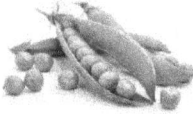

For a hungry man, green peas are shinier than gleaming pearls. ~Lenard Stewart

Gracious Green Peas

Lowers cholesterol

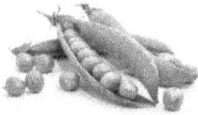

Cancer fighter

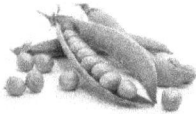

Supports cardiovascular system

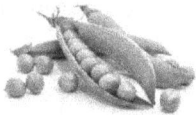

High in antioxidants

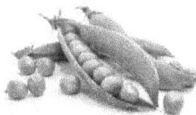

Anti-inflammatory

Health Benefits of Green Peas

Daily consumption of green beans is among the main food groups for preventing disease and optimizing health. Green peas are a valuable source of fiber. Green peas promote intestinal health by binding to cholesterol and helping to excrete it. They also maintain stable energy by slowing down the appearance of glucose in the blood.

High in Anti-Oxidants

Green peas are an excellent source of phytonutrients with anti-oxidant activity. The antioxidants in green peas help in decreasing cardiovascular disease and later help to reduce the risk of heart disease and stroke.

Stabilize Blood Pressure

Green peas can help lower high blood pressure and protect against heart disease.

Promotes Proper Cell Formation

Green peas help propel activity that creates proper blood cell formation.

High Source of Dietary Fiber

Green peas are a source of dietary fiber which helps keep the digestive tract in check. Fiber acts to prevent constipation and other gastro-intestinal issues.

Sweetest Sweet Potatoes

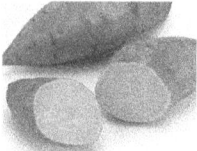

My dream is to become a farmer, just a Bohemian guy pulling up his own sweet potatoes for dinner. ~ Lenny Kravitz

Sweetest Sweet Potatoes

Saves your eyesight

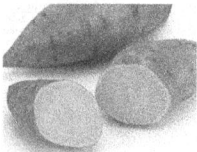

Lifts mood

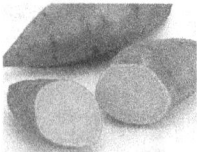

Combats cancer

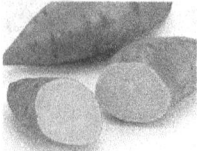

Strengthens bones

Health Benefits of Sweet Potatoes
The consumption of sweet potatoes helps play an important role in bone and tooth formation, digestion, and blood cell formation. Sweet potatoes help accelerate wound healing through promoting the production of collagen which helps maintain skin's youthful elasticity.

Promotes Proper Cell Formation
The consumption of sweet potatoes promotes proper red and white blood cell production and helps metabolize protein.

Healthy Nerve Function
Sweet potatoes promote healthy arteries, blood, bone, heart, muscle, and nerve function.

Relax Muscle Contractions

Sweet potatoes help regulate heartbeat and nerve signals. Sweet potatoes help relax muscle contractions, reducing swelling, and help protect the activity of the kidneys.

Regulate Blood Sugar

Sweet potatoes have natural sugars that are slowly released into the bloodstream, helping to ensure a balanced and regular source of energy, without the blood sugar spikes

Precious Pumpkins

Pumpkin pie, if rightly made, is a thing of beauty and a joy - while it lasts. ~ The House Mother.

Precious Pumpkins

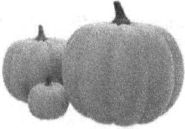

Antioxidant rich

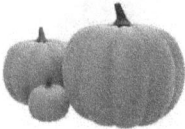

Helps hydrate the body

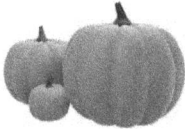

Lowers risk for hypertension

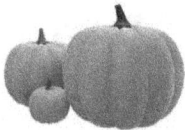

Supports bone density

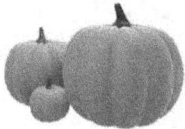

Boosts immune system

Health Benefits of Pumpkins

Pumpkin has been known to cure wounds and treat burns. Ingesting pumpkin along with the seeds promotes kidney and urinary tract support. Pumpkin is beneficial in ridding the body of intestinal worms.

Antioxidant Rich

The rich orange color, the flavonoids and the phytonutrients in pumpkin promotes the systems of the body to be less likely to develop certain cancers.

Regulate Blood Pressure

The nutrients in pumpkin help lower the risk for hypertension through regulation of blood pressure.

Strengthen the Immune System

The antioxidants in pumpkins are known to strengthen our immune system that lowers the potential risk of immune suppressant diseases.

Healthy Skin

Intake of pumpkin is helpful in maintaining the integrity of skin and mucus membranes. The antioxidants in pumpkin also promote healthy lungs and oral cavity.

Stabilizes Cholesterol

Pumpkins contain powerful antioxidants that are known as anti-inflammatory agents. These antioxidants help prevent a build-up of cholesterol on the arterial walls; this in turn lowers the chance of stroke.

Synchronizes Bowel Movements

The high fiber content of pumpkin helps promote a healthy digestive system. Ingesting pumpkins leads to synchronized bowel movements that help to remove toxins from the body.

Radiant Radishes

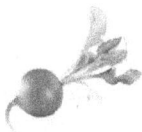

Radishes are like small pepper pots with a beautiful shiny glaze. ~D. Francis

Radiant Radishes

Detoxifies the body

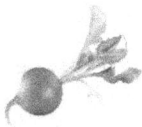

Alleviates constipation

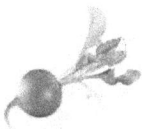

Supports healthy kidney and liver

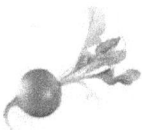

Anticancer

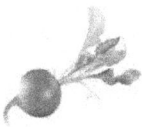

Anti-inflammatory

Radiant Radishes

Radishes are great for the liver and the stomach. It acts as a detoxifier that purifies the blood. Radishes also promote the production of red blood cells by increasing supply of fresh oxygen in the blood.

Rich in Fiber

Radish is rich in fiber. This fiber facilitates digestion, retains water and helps ease constipation. Being a great detoxifier, it helps to heal and soothe the digestive and excretory system.

Urinary Tract Health
Radishes are diuretic in nature which increases urine production. Radish also helps alleviate inflammation of the urinary tract. It also cleans the kidneys and inhibits infections in kidneys and urinary system.

Healthy Skin
The water in radishes help maintain moisture in the skin. Smashed raw radish can act as a facial cleanser. Due to its disinfectant properties, radish is helpful in refreshing drying skin, rashes and cracks.

Healthy Kidneys
Radishes are considered as a diuretic, a cleanser and a disinfectant. Its diuretic properties help wash away the toxins accumulated in the kidneys. Cleansing properties lessen accumulation of toxins in the blood. Its disinfectant properties also help protect the kidneys.

Regulate Body Temperature
Radishes help bring down the body temperature and relieve inflammation due to fever.

Health Repertory System
Radish is an anti-congestive; it relieves congestion of respiratory system including nose, throat, wind-pipe and lungs, due to cold, infection, allergies and other causes of infections.

Superior Spinach

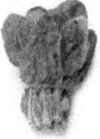

Green, Bountiful and Precious Spinach. ~ Cooking is an Art

Superior Spinach

Anticancer agent

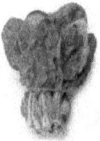

Supports cardiovascular health

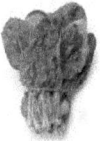

Stabilizes blood sugar

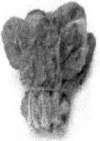

Alleviates constipation

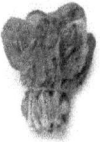

Alleviates anemia

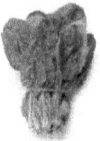

Aids digestion

Health Benefits of Spinach
Spinach is a nutrient-dense food. The phytonutrients in spinach help to prevent thickening and hardening of arteries. Spinach also helps to stabilize blood sugar among diabetics. Spinach is loaded with flavonoids that function as antioxidants and anti-cancer agents.

Healthy Heart
Spinach is a heart-healthy food. The antioxidants in spinach help reduce free radical amounts in the body. The antioxidants work to keep cholesterol from oxidizing.

Gastrointestinal Health
Spinach protects the cells of the body's colon from the harmful effects of free radicals. Also, DNA damage and mutations in colon cells may be prevented by ingesting spinach daily.

Anti-inflammatory Properties
Spinach has anti-inflammatory properties that help to alleviate inflammation throughout the body.

Brain Power
Consumption of spinach may slow age-related decline in brain function and agility.

Why Take Whole Food Supplements? Juice Plus+ The Next Best Thing to Fruits and Vegetables

Juice Plus+ really is a great, easy, and inexpensive step you can take in the right direction. That's true not only in terms of the added whole food based nutrition it provides, but also because of its demonstrated ability to help "jumpstart" both children and adults into making other healthy changes. ~The Juice Plus+ Guide To Better Health

The recommended amount of fruits and vegetables needed to be ingested daily according to USDA is 9 to 13 servings. Now we have discussed the wide array of health benefits of eating fruits and vegetables to heal the body and prevent future disease.

We know that principal benefit of ingestion of antioxidants seems to stem from the consumption of a wide array of phytonutrients from fruits and vegetables. This is why whole food supplements that contain a combination of plant compounds acting together may provide more benefits than individual isolated vitamins alone.

Juice Plus+ is created by dehydrating and concentrating a variety of fruits, vegetables and whole grains and then encapsulating them.

Juice Plus+ may be an option for people who would like to take advantage of the health benefits of fruits and vegetables in your daily diet. **For more information on the benefits of Juice Plus visit:** http://Deborah.JuicePlus.com/ http://Deborah.TowerGarden.com

Top Antioxidant Fruits

Researchers at the Human Nutrition Research Center on Aging at Tufts University figured it out by measuring various fruits and vegetables for their ORAC (oxygen radical absorbance capacity), antioxidant power.

*Prunes *Raisins *Blueberries *Blackberries *Strawberries *Raspberries *Plums *Oranges *Red Grapes *Cherries

Top Antioxidant Vegetables

*Kale *Spinach *Brussel Sprouts *Alfalfa Sprouts *Broccoli *Beets *Red Bell Peppers *Onions *Corn *Eggplant

Top Fruits and Vegetables to get Iron High in Iron

Fruits and vegetables that contain 3.6 mg or more iron per reference amount (20% of the Daily Value per reference amount) qualify to carry the label "high in iron." Examples include:

*Lentils *Spinach *White Beans *Winged Beans *Dried Apricots *Chickpeas *Green Soybeans *Lima Beans *Pigeon Peas *Pink Beans *Pinto Beans *Small White Beans

Top Brain Enhancing Foods – Foods that make you feel good!

*Blueberries *Strawberries *Blackberries *Banana
*Avocado *Tomatoes *Broccoli *Red Cabbage *Spinach
*Eggplant

Top High Protein Fruits and Vegetables

(Yes you most definitely get all the protein you need from fruits and vegetables)

Food	Grams of Protein
Almonds (3oz.)	10
Banana (1)	1.2
Broccoli (2 cups)	10
Brown rice (1cup)	5
Chickpeas (1 cup)	15
Corn (1 cup)	4.2
Lentils (1cup)	18
Green Peas (1 cup)	7
Tofu (4 ounces)	11
Kidney Beans (1 cup)	14

Top High Calcium Fruits and Vegetables

Food	Calcium Content
Kale (1cup)	449 mg
Bok Choy (1cup)	787 mg
Broccoli (1cup)	189 mg
Orange (2)	120mg
Raisins (1/2 cup)	60mg
Soybeans (1cup)	261 mg
Spinach (1 cup)	244 mg
Tofu (1cup)	300mg
Collard Greens (1 cup)	350mg

Top Fruits and Vegetables that Prevent Diabetes

*Beans *Spinach *Collards *Kale *Grapefruit *Oranges
*Lemons *Sweet Potatoes   *Berries *Tomatoes

Top Fruits and Vegetables that Prevent Cancer

*Garlic *Spinach *Collards *Kale *Grapes *Tomatoes *Blueberries *Cabbage *Broccoli *Cauliflower

Top Fruits and Vegetables that Prevent Hypertension

*Lemon *Orange *Apple *Prunes *Asparagus *Beets *Broccoli *Cabbage *Carrots *Celery

Top Fruits and Vegetables that Prevent Heart Disease

*Berries *Pear *Romaine *lettuce *Cucumber *Spinach *Kale *Tomatoes *Beans *Radish *Onions

Top Fruits and Vegetables that Boost Immunity

*Oranges *Grapefruit *Lemon *Cauliflower *Carrots *Kale *Mushrooms *Watermelon *Garlic *Apples

References and Sources:

This book is a compilation of research available online and off line of many specified and documented reports. It is not meant as a medical opinion and accuracy of information has not been independently verified.

Apples

Barbosa AC, Pinto MD, Sarkar D et al. Varietal Influences on Antihyperglycemia Properties of Freshly Harvested Apples Using In Vitro Assay Models. J Med Food. 2010 Sep 27. [Epub ahead of print] 2010.

Bazzano LA, He J, Ogden LG, Loria CM, Whelton PK. Dietary fiber intake and reduced risk of coronary heart disease in US men and women: the National Health and Nutrition Examination Survey I Epidemiologic Follow-up Study. Arch Intern Med. 2003 Sep 8;163(16):1897-904 2003.

Huxley RR, Neil HAW. The relation between dietary flavonol intake and coronary heart disease mortality: a meta-analysis of prospective cohort studies. European Journal of Clinical Nutrition (2003) 57, 904-908. 2003

Apricot

Jian L, Lee AH, Binns CW. Tea and lycopene protect against prostate cancer. Asia Pac J Clin Nutr. 2007;16 Suppl 1:453-7. 2007. PMID:17392149.

Wills RB, Scriven FM, Greenfield H. Nutrient composition of stone fruit (Prunus spp.) cultivars: apricot, cherry, nectarine, peach and plum. J Sci Food Agric 1983 Dec;34(12):1383-9 1983. PMID:16280.

Bananas

Bazzano LA, He J, Ogden LG, Loria CM, Whelton PK. Dietary fiber intake and reduced risk of coronary heart disease in US men and women: the National Health and Nutrition Examination Survey I Epidemiologic Follow-up Study. Arch Intern Med. 2003 Sep 8;163(16):1897-904   2003.

Rabbani GH, Teka T, Saha SK, Zaman B, Majid N, Khatun M, Wahed MA, Fuchs GJ. Green banana and pectin improve small intestinal permeability and reduce fluid loss in Bangladeshi children with persistent diarrhea. Dig Dis

Rao NM. Protease inhibitors from ripened and unripe Ned bananas. Biochem Int 1991 May; 24(1):13-22 1991.

Blackberries

"Journal of the American Medical Association"; Content of Redox-Active Compounds (ie, antioxidants) in Foods Consumed in the United States; Bente L Halvorsen, et al; July 2006

The New Healing Herbs"; Michael Castleman; 2001

Wang SY, Lin HS. Antioxidant activity in fruits and leaves of blackberry, raspberry, and strawberry varies with cultivar and developmental stage. J Agric Food Chem 2000 Feb;48(2):140-6 2000. PMID:13820.

Black Currant

Complete Book of Food Counts"; Corrinne Netzer 2009

McKinley Health Center; "Macronutrients: The Importance of Carbohydrate, Protein and Fat"; March 2008

Blueberries

Vuong T, Matar C, Ramassamy C et al. Biotransformed blueberry juice protects neurons from hydrogen peroxide-induced oxidative stress and mitogen-activated protein kinase pathway alterations. Br J Nutr. 2010 Sep;104(5):656-63. Epub 2010 May 12. 2010.

Wang SY, Chen CT, Sciarappa W et al. Fruit quality, antioxidant capacity, and flavonoid content of organically and conventionally grown blueberries. J Agric Food Chem. 2008 Jul 23;56(14):5788-94. Epub 2008 Jul 1. 2008.

Wang SY, Lin HS. Antioxidant activity in fruits and leaves of blackberry, raspberry, and strawberry varies with cultivar and developmental stage. J Agric Food Chem 2000 Feb;48(2):140-6 2000. PMID:13820.

Cantaloupe
Khaw KT, Bingham S, Welch A, et al. Relation between plasma ascorbic acid and mortality in men and women in EPIC-Norfolk prospective study: a prospective population study. European Prospective Investigation into Cancer and Nutrition. Lancet. 2001 Mar 3;357(9257):657-63 2001.

Lamikanra O. Keeping Just-Cut Cantaloupe Fresh and Flavorful. Food and Nutrition Research Briefs, USDA Agricultural Research Service, October 2005 2005.

Cherry
Oregon Health and Science University: Tart Cherry Juice Reduces Muscle Pain and Inflammation; July 7, 2010

Behavioral Brain Research"; Tart Cherry Anthocyanins Suppress Inflammation-induced Pain Behavior in Rats; Tall et al.; 2004

Coconut

British Journal of Cancer"; A Comparison of Long-Chain Triglycerides and Medium-Chain Triglycerides on Weight Loss and Tumor Size in a Cachexia Model; M.J. Tisdale, et al.; November 1988

MayoClinic.com; Can coconut oil help me lose weight?; Katherine Zeratsky, R.D., L.D.; Aug. 2010

Cranberries

MayoClinic.com: Dietary Fiber: Essential for a Healthy Diet

"Critical Reviews in Food Science and Nutrition"; Cranberry Flavonoids, Atherosclerosis and Cardiovascular Health; Reed J; January 2002

Fig

Rubnov S, Kashman Y, Rabinowitz R, et al. Suppressors of cancer cell proliferation from fig (Ficus carica) resin: isolation and structure elucidation. J Nat Prod 2001 Jul;64(7):993-6 2001. PMID:13390.

Serraclara A, Hawkins F, Perez C, et al. Hypoglycemic action of an oral fig-leaf decoction in type-I diabetic patients. Diabetes Res Clin Pract 1998 Jan;39(1):19-22 1998. PMID:13430.

Grapes

Yadav M, Jain S, Bhardwaj A et al. Biological and medicinal properties of grapes and their bioactive constituents: an update. J Med Food. 2009 Jun;12(3):473-84. Review. 2009.

Zamyatnin AA and Voronina OL. Antimicrobial and other oligopeptides of grapes. Biochemistry (Mosc). 2010 Feb;75(2):214-23. 2010.

Zunino S. Type 2 diabetes and glycemic response to grapes or grape products. J Nutr. 2009 Sep;139(9):1794S-800S. Epub 2009 Jul 22. Review. 2009.

Grapefruit

Mahan LK, Stump S. Krause's Food Nutrition and Diet Therapy 10th Ed. WB Saunders Co 2000 2000.

Matos HR, Di Mascio P, Medeiros MH. Protective effect of lycopene on lipid peroxidation and oxidative DNA damage in cell culture. Arch Biochem Biophys 2000 Nov 1;383(1):56-9 2000.

Lemon

Kawaii S, Tomono Y, Katase E, et al. Antiproliferative effects of the readily extractable fractions prepared from various citrus juices on several cancer cell lines. J Agric Food Chem 1999 Jul;47(7):2509-12 1999. PMID:13190.

Mango

Purdue University: Mango

National Mango Board: Mango Nutrition

Nectarine

Produce for Better Health Foundation: Nectarine -- Nutrition, Selection, Storage

US Food and Drug Administration: 9. Appendix A -- Definitions of Nutrient Content Claims

Oranges

Galati EM, Monforte MT, Kirjavainen S, et al. Biological effects of hesperidin, a citrus flavonoid. (Note I): antiinflammatory and analgesic activity. Farmaco 1994 Nov;40(11):709-12 1994. PMID:13070.

Guarnieri S, Riso P, Porrini M. Orange juice vs vitamin C: effect on hydrogen peroxide-induced DNA damage in mononuclear blood cells. Br J Nutr. 2007 Apr;97(4):639-43. 2007. PMID:17349075.

Yuan JM, Stram DO, Arakawa K, Lee HP, Yu MC. Dietary cryptoxanthin and reduced risk of lung cancer: the Singapore Chinese

Health Study. Cancer Epidemiol Biomarkers Prev. 2003 Sep;12(9):890-8. 2003.

Peaches

Mayo Clinic: Treating Anemia Can Boost Energy
Colorado State University: Dietary Fiber

Pears

Ensminger AH, Esminger M. K. J. e. al. Food for Health: A Nutrition Encyclopedia. Clovis, California: Pegus Press; 1986 1986. PMID:15210.

Pineapples

The Queensland Institute of Medical Research,. Pineapple stems that show anti-tumor activity. Medical Research News, July 19, 2005.

Plums

Nakatani N, Kayano S, Kikuzaki H, et al. Identification, quantitative determination, and antioxidative activities of chlorogenic acid isomers in prune (Prunus domestica L.). J Agric Food Chem 2000 Nov;48(11):5512-6 2000. PMID:13580.

Strawberries

Liu M, Li XQ, Weber C et al. Antioxidant and antiproliferative activities of raspberries. J Agric Food Chem 2002 May 8;50(10):2926-30 2002.

Wang SY, Lin HS. Antioxidant activity in fruits and leaves of blackberry, raspberry, and strawberry varies with cultivar and developmental stage. J Agric Food Chem 2000 Feb;48(2):140-6 2000. PMID:13820.

Seeram NP, Momin RA, Nair MG, Bourquin LD. Cyclooxygenase inhibitory and antioxidant cyanidin glycosides in cherries and berries. Phytomedicine 2001 Sep;8(5):362-9 2001. PMID:13780.

Tomatoes

Silaste ML, Alfthan G, Aro A, et al. Tomato juice decreases LDL cholesterol levels and increases LDL resistance to oxidation. Br J Nutr. 2007 Dec;98(6):1251-8. 2007. PMID:17617941

Tan HL, Thomas-Ahner JM, Grainger EM et al. Tomato-based food products for prostate cancer prevention: what have we learned? . Cancer Metastasis Rev. 2010 Sep;29(3):553-68. 2010.

Willcox JK, Catignani GL, Lazarus S. Tomatoes and cardiovascular health. Crit Rev Food Sci Nutr 2003;43(1):1-18 2003.

Watermelon
Edwards AJ, Vineyard BT, Wiley ER et al. Consumption of watermelon juice increases plasma concentrations of lycopene and beta-carotene in humans. J Nutr 2003 Apr;133(4):1043-50 2003.

Vegetables

Argula
Linus Pauling Institute at Oregon State University: Micronutrient Information Center: Cruciferous Vegetables (Web)

Mutation Research"; Cancer-Preventive Isothiocyanates: Measurement of Human Exposure and Mechanism of Action; Y. Zhang; November 2004 (Web)

Nutrition and You; Arugula (Salad Rocket) Nutrition Facts and Health Benefits (Web)

Asparagus
Shao Y, Chin CK, Ho CT et al. Anti-tumor activity of the crude saponins obtained from asparagus. Cancer Lett. 1996 Jun 24;104(1):31-6. 1996.

Sidiq T, Khajuria A, Suden P et al. A novel sarsasapogenin glycoside from Asparagus racemosus elicits protective immune responses against HBsAg. Immunol Lett. 2011 Mar 30;135(1-2):129-35. Epub 2010 Oct 28. 2011.

Avacado
Rosenblat G, Meretski S, Segal J et al. Polyhydroxylated fatty alcohols derived from avocado suppresses inflammatory response and provides non-sunscreen protection against UV-induced damage in skin cells. Arch Dermatol Res. 2010 Oct 27. [Epub ahead of print]. 2010.

Unlu NZ, Bohn T, Clinton SK et al. Carotenoid Absorption from Salad and Salsa by Humans Is Enhanced by the Addition of Avocado or Avocado Oil. J. Nutr., Mar 2005; 135: 431 - 436. 2005.

Brocolli
Li F, Hullar MAJ, Schwarz Y, et al. Human Gut Bacterial Communities Are Altered by Addition of Cruciferous Vegetables to a Controlled Fruit- and Vegetable-Free Diet. Journal of Nutrition, Vol. 139, No. 9, 1685-1691, September 2009.

Vasanthi HR, Mukherjee S and Das DK. Potential health benefits of broccoli- a chemical-biological overview. Mini Rev Med Chem. 2009 Jun;9(6):749-59. 2009.

Cabbage
Ambrosone CB, Tang L. Cruciferous vegetable intake and cancer prevention: role of nutrigenetics. Cancer Prev Res (Phila Pa). 2009 Apr;2(4):298-300. 2009.

Kusznierewicz, B, Bartoszek A., Wolska, L et al. Partial characterization of white cabbages (Brassica oleracea var. capitata f. alba) from different regions by glucosinolates, bioactive compounds, total antioxidant activities, and proteins. LWT Food Science and Technology 2008, 41, 1-9. 2008.

Carrots

Lin BH and Lucier G. . Carrot Consumption Varies With Age, Income, and Race. Amber Waves. Washington: Apr 2008. Vol. 6, Iss. 2; p. 4. 2008.

Soltoft M, Bysted A, Madsen KH et al. Effects of organic and conventional growth systems on the content of carotenoids in carrot roots, and on intake and plasma status of carotenoids in humans. J Sci Food Agric. 2011 Mar 15;91(4):767-75. doi: 10.1002/jsfa.4248. Epub 2011 Jan 6. 2011.

Cauliflower

Nettleton JA, Steffen LM, Mayer-Davis EJ, et al. Dietary patterns are associated with biochemical markers of inflammation and endothelial activation in the Multi-Ethnic Study of Atherosclerosis (MESA). Am J Clin Nutr. 2006 Jun;83(6):1369-79. 2006.

Celery

University of Maryland Medical Center: Celery Seed
Texas A&M Horticulture Department: Celery First Used as a Medicine

Collard Greens

Li F, Hullar MAJ, Schwarz Y, et al. Human Gut Bacterial Communities Are Altered by Addition of Cruciferous Vegetables to a Controlled Fruit- and Vegetable-Free Diet. Journal of Nutrition, Vol. 139, No. 9, 1685-1691, September 2009.

Corn

Kwon YI, Apostolidis E, Kim YC et al. Health benefits of traditional corn, beans, and pumpkin: in vitro studies for hyperglycemia and hypertension management. J Med Food. 2007 Jun;10(2):266-75. 2007.

Cucumber

Rios JL, Recio MC, Escandell JM, et al. Inhibition of transcription factors by plant-derived compounds and their implications in inflammation and cancer. Curr Pharm Des. 2009;15(11):1212-37. Review. 2009.

Tang J, Meng X, Liu H et al. Antimicrobial activity of sphingolipids isolated from the stems of cucumber (Cucumis sativus L.). Molecules. 2010 Dec 15;15(12):9288-97. 2010

Eggplant
Noda Y, Kneyuki T, Igarashi K, et al. Antioxidant activity of nasunin, an anthocyanin in eggplant peels. Toxicology 2000 Aug 7;148(2-3):119-23 2000.

Lettuce (Romaine)
Produce for Better Health Foundation: Fruits and Veggies More Matters: Romaine Lettuce Nutrition Information (Web)

"The Washington Post"; Romaine's Long, Leafy History; Barbara Damrosch; February 2008

Mushroom
Yarnell E and Abascal K. Holistic Approaches to Prostate Cancer. Alternative & Complementary Therapies, Volume 14, Number 4 (August 2008), pp. 164-180. 2008.

Onions
Wilson EA and Demmig-Adams B. Antioxidant, anti-inflammatory, and antimicrobial properties of garlic and onions. Nutrition & Food Science 2007, Vol. 37 Iss: 3, pp.178 - 183. 2007.

Yang J, Meyers KJ, van der Heide J, Liu RH. Varietal Differences in Phenolic Content and Antioxidant and Antiproliferative Activities of Onions. J Agric Food Chem. 2004 Nov 3;52(22):6787-6793. 2004. PMID:15506817.

Peas (Green)
Sievenpiper JL, Kendall CW, Esfahani A et al. Effect of non-oil-seed pulses on glycaemic control: a systematic review and meta-analysis of randomised controlled experimental trials in people with and without diabetes. Diabetologia. 2009 Aug;52(8):1479-95. 2009.

Pumpkin
Jayaprakasam B, Seeram NP, Nair MG. Anticancer and anti-inflammatory activities of cucurbitaceous from Cucurbita andreana. Cancer Lett 2003 Jan 10;189(1):11-6 2003.

Radishes
USDA Nutrient Database: Nutrient Data Laboratory (Web) Harvard School of Public Health: Fiber -- Start Roughing It (Web) Harvard School of Public Health: Protein -- Moving Closer to Center Stage (Web)

Sweet Potatoes
Mei X, Mu TH and Han JJ. Composition and physicochemical properties of dietary fiber extracted from residues of 10 varieties of sweet potato by a sieving method. J Agric Food Chem. 2010 Jun 23;58(12):7305-10. 2010.

Xie J, Han YT, Wang CB et al. Purple sweet potato pigments protect murine thymocytes from (60)Co gamma-ray-induced mitochondria-mediated apoptosis. Int J Radiat Biol. 2010 Aug 10. [Epub ahead of print] 2010.

Spinach
Longnecker MP, Newcomb PA, Mittendorf R, et al. Intake of carrots, spinach, and supplements containing vitamin A in relation to risk of breast cancer. Cancer Epidemiol Biomarkers Prev 1997 Nov;6(11):887-92 1997. PMID:12980.

Morris MC, Evans DA, Tangney CC, Bienias JL, Wilson RS. Associations of vegetable and fruit consumption with age-related cognitive change. Neurology. 2006 Oct 24;67(8):1370-6. 2006. PMID:17060562.

Wang Y, Chang CF, Chou J, Chen HL, Deng X, Harvey BK, Cadet JL, Bickford PC. Dietary supplementation with blueberries, spinach, or spirulina reduces ischemic brain damage. Exp Neurol. 2005 May;193(1):75-84. 2005. PMID:15817266.

Recommended Websites

The List Below provides a number of other resources that you can use to learn more about the subject of health wellness.

Juice Plus+ Whole Food Supplement

Deborah Francis

http://Deborah.JuicePlus.com/

Facts about Juice Plus+

www.juiceplusfacts.com

Children's Health Study

www.childrenshealthstudy.com

The Worlds Healthiest Foods

www.whfoods.com

Dr. Mercola (World Renowedened Naturopathic Doctor)

http://articles.mercola.com/sites/current.aspx

Dr. Sears (World Renowned Pediatrician)

www.askdrsears.com/

Dr. Mitra Ray (World Renowned Natural Health Researcher)

www.drmitraray.com/

American Academy of Pediatrics

www.aap.org

American Cancer Society

www.cancer.org

American College of Sports Medicine

www.excersciseismedicine.org

American Council on Exercise

www.acefitness.org/getfit

American Heart Association

www.americanheart.org

American Heart Association's Go Red for Women

www.goredforwomen.org

Arthritis Foundation

www.arthritis.org

www.letsmovetogether.org

Centers for Disease Control and Prevention

www.cdc.gov

www.fruitsandveggiesmatter.gov

www.bam.gov

Department of Health and Human Services

www.smallstep.gov

Eat Smart Play Hard Healthy Lifestyle (USDA)

http://www.fns.usda.gov/eatsmartplayhardhealthylifestyle/

Health Canada: Food and Nutrition

http://www.hc-sc.gc.ca/fn-an/index-eng.php

Healthier US (Department of Health and Human Services)

www.healthierUS.gov

National Coalition for Promoting Physical Activity

www.ncppa.org

National Institutes of Health

www.nib.gov

Nutrition Detectives

www.nutitiondetectives.com

The American Diabetes Association

www.diabetes.org

The President's Council on Physical Fiteness

www.fitness.gov

United States Department of Agriculture

www.mypyramid.gov